NEW FUNCTIONAL TRAINING FOR SPORTS

Second Edition

Michael Boyle

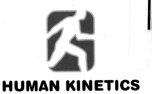

HUMAN KINETICS

Library of Congress Cataloging-in-Publication Data

Names: Boyle, Michael, 1959- author.
Title: New functional training for sports / Michael Boyle.
Other titles: Functional training for sports
Description: Second Edition. | Champaign, IL : Human Kinetics, [2016] |
  Includes index.
Identifiers: LCCN 2016002990 (print) | LCCN 2016020908 (ebook) | ISBN
  9781492530619 (print) | ISBN 9781492530626 (ebook)
Subjects: LCSH: Athletes--Training of. | Physical education and training. |
  Exercise.
Classification: LCC GV711.5 .B69 2016 (print) | LCC GV711.5 (ebook) | DDC
  796.07--dc23
LC record available at https://lccn.loc.gov/2016002990

ISBN: 978-1-4925-3061-9 (print)

This publication is written and published to provide accurate and authoritative information relevant to the subject matter presented. It is published and sold with the understanding that the author and publisher are not engaged in rendering legal, medical, or other professional services by reason of their authorship or publication of this work. If medical or other expert assistance is required, the services of a competent professional person should be sought.

The web addresses cited in this text were current as of February 2016, unless otherwise noted.

Developmental Editor: Kevin Matz; **Senior Managing Editor:** Elizabeth Evans; **Copyeditor:** Patricia MacDonald; **Indexer:** Laurel Plotzke; **Senior Graphic Designer:** Joe Buck; **Graphic Designer:** Tara Welsch; **Cover Designer:** Keith Blomberg; **Photograph (cover):** © Human Kinetics; **Photographs (interior):** © Human Kinetics, unless otherwise noted; **Video Producer:** Doug Fink; **Photo Asset Manager:** Laura Fitch; **Visual Production Assistant:** Joyce Brumfield; **Photo Production Manager:** Jason Allen; **Art Manager:** Kelly Hendren; **Illustrations:** © Human Kinetics; **Printer:** Walsworth

We thank Mike Boyle Strength and Conditioning in Woburn, MA, for assistance in providing the location for the photo shoot for this book.

Human Kinetics books are available at special discounts for bulk purchase. Special editions or book excerpts can also be created to specification. For details, contact the Special Sales Manager at Human Kinetics.

Printed in the United States of America   10 9 8 7

The paper in this book was manufactured using responsible forestry methods.

Human Kinetics
P.O. Box 5076
Champaign, IL 61825-5076
Website: www.HumanKinetics.com

In the United States, email info@hkusa.com or call 800-747-4457.
In Canada, email info@hkcanada.com.
In the United Kingdom/Europe, email hk@hkeurope.com.

For information about Human Kinetics' coverage in other areas of the world,
please visit our website: **www.HumanKinetics.com**

E6784

CONTENTS

iii

VIDEO CONTENTS

Foam Rolling, Stretching, and Dynamic Warm-Up

Foam Rolling the Gluteus Maximus and Hip Rotators

Foam Rolling the Low Back

Foam Rolling the Upper Back

Foam Rolling the Tensor Fasciae Latae and Gluteus Medius

Foam Rolling the Adductors

Foam Rolling the Posterior Shoulder

Foam Rolling the Pecs

Box Hip Flexor Stretch

T-Spine Drill 2

T-Spine Drill 3

Ankle Mobility Drill 1

Ankle Mobility Drill 2

Hip Mobility Drill 2

Hip Mobility Drill 3

Floor Slides

Backward Lunge Walk With Hamstring Stretch

Backward Straight-Leg Deadlift Walk

Straight-Leg Skip

Lateral Skip

Cross-Over Skip

Carioca

Lateral Crawl

Shuffle Wide and Stick

Shuffle Quick and Stick

Cross in Front

In-In-Out-Out

Scissors

Hip Switch

Lower Body Training

Kettlebell Swings

Split Squat

Slide-Board Lunge

Cross-Reaching Single-Leg Straight-Leg Deadlift

Cable Loaded Single-Leg Straight-Leg Deadlift

Stability Ball Leg Curl

Core Training

Stability Ball Rollout

Body Saw

Ab Wheel Rollout

Half-Kneeling In-Line Stable Chop

Half-Kneeling In-Line Stable Lift

Lunge-Position Chop

Standing Chop

Standing Lift

Standing Transverse Chop

Step-Up Lift

Get-Ups

Medicine Ball Side Throw

Medicine Ball Half-Kneeling Side-Twist Throw

Medicine Ball Front-Twist Throw

Medicine Ball Single-Leg Front-Twist Throw

Medicine Ball Standing Overhead Throw

Medicine Ball Tall Kneeling Chest Throw

Upper Body Training

Cat–Cow
Single-Arm Double-Leg
   Rotational Throw
Sports Flex High-Low
Sports Flex T
Standing External Rotation

Plyometric Training

Total Gym Jump Trainer
Box Jump
Single-Leg Box Hop
Single-Leg Lateral Box Hop
Lateral Bound and Stick
Hurdle Jump and Stick
Single-Leg Hurdle Hop and
   Stick
Single-Leg Lateral Hurdle
   Hop and Stick
45-Degree Bound and Stick
45-Degree Lateral Bound
Power Skip

Olympic Lifting

Hang Clean
Close-Grip Snatch
Single-Arm Dumbbell Snatch
Single-Leg Clean or Single-
   Leg Snatch

ACCESSING THE ONLINE VIDEO

This book includes access to online video that includes 71 clips demonstrating many of the exercises found in the book. Throughout the book, exercises marked with this play button icon indicate where the content is enhanced by online video clips.

   Take the following steps to access the video. If you need help at any point in the process, you can contact us by clicking on the Technical Support link under Customer Service on the right side of the screen.

1. Visit www.HumanKinetics.com/NewFunctionalTrainingforSports.
2. Click on the **View online video** link next to the book cover.
3. You will be directed to the screen in figure 1. Click the **Sign In** link on the left or top of the page. If you do not have an account with Human Kinetics, you will be prompted to create one.

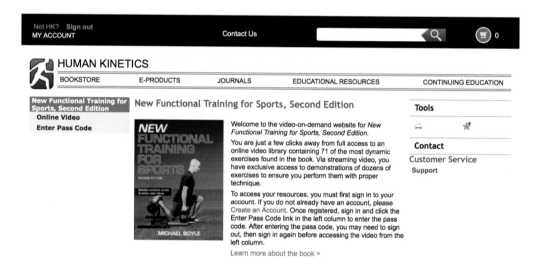

Figure 1

4. If the online video does not appear in the list on the left of the page, click the **Enter Pass Code** option in that list. Enter the pass code that is printed here, including all hyphens. Click the **Submit** button to unlock the online video. After you have entered this pass code the first time, you will never have to enter it again. For future visits, all you need to do is sign in to the book's website and follow the link that appears in the left menu.

Pass code for online video: BOYLE-9NXR-OV

5. Once you have signed into the site and entered the pass code, select **Online Video** from the list on the left side of the screen. You'll then see an Online Video page with information about the video, as shown in figure 2. You can go straight to the accompanying videos for each topic by clicking on the blue links at the bottom of the page.

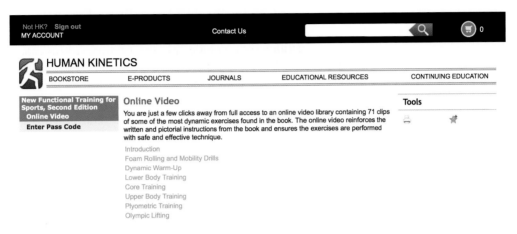

Figure 2

6. You are now able to view video for the topic you selected on the previous screen, as well as others that accompany this product. Across the top of the page, you will see a set of buttons that correspond to the topics in the text that have accompanying video:
   - Foam Rolling and Mobility Drills
   - Dynamic Warm-Up
   - Lower Body Training
   - Core Training
   - Upper Body Training
   - Plyometric Training
   - Olympic Lifting

7. Once you click on a topic, a player will appear. In the player, the clips for that topic will appear vertically along the right side. Select the video you would like to watch and view it in the main player window. You can use the buttons at the bottom of the main player window to view the video full screen, to turn captioning on and off, and to pause, fast-forward, or reverse the clip.

FOREWORD

Unqualified was the word that most loudly reverberated through my head when Michael asked me to write a foreword for this book. I know little of the pioneers in strength and conditioning. And I've given no more than a cursory sift through the many physical training publications.

However, upon further reflection, maybe I had sold myself short. Maybe this strength and conditioning neophyte was exactly the person qualified to evaluate the expertise and insight of Michael Boyle's functional training programs. After all, who better to validate Michael's vast knowledge and methods than an athlete who trained under his tutelage?

I have been a professional baseball player for 14 years and spent the last 9 in the major leagues. I have been traded and released, injured and healthy. I have won two World Series, and I've finished in last place. There is very little I have not seen, and even less I have not heard.

I entered the world of professional baseball at a time when players were members of one of two classes. There was the position player, or athlete, as distinct from the pitcher, or nonathlete. Position players trained for strength gains, striving to replicate the masses of bodybuilders. Pitchers ran poles. Over the past decade we have seen a paradigm shift in how we approach functional training. Pitchers are considered athletes (gasp), and athletes train to be athletic.

Michael Boyle has been a trendsetter in his dynamic approach to strength and conditioning, incorporating components of therapy, flexibility, stability, strength, and power to his workouts. I know, because I spent the winter of 2014 at the Michael Boyle Strength and Conditioning facility.

Michael and I met in 2012 when I was traded to the Boston Red Sox. He was working as a strength and conditioning consultant for the organization. A couple of brief conversations left me impressed. So I thumbed through the original edition of Michael's *Advances in Functional Training* and was even more inspired. His approach made sense to me. In the preface of that book, Mike referred to a friend who had concisely described a proper training workout as one in which an athlete is required to "push something, pull something and do something with your legs." The simplicity of that statement struck a chord. For my functional training program, I would amend the phrase only slightly to "lift something, throw something against the wall, and jump over something."

Through the years, Michael and I have shared thoughtful dialogue about pitching mechanics, injury prevention, and velocity creation. I have witnessed Michael learn, concurrent with watching him educate. Indeed, at his core, Michael is a teacher. And a very fine one at that.

However, what distinguishes Michael in this industry is his ability to clearly communicate the physiology and kinesiology underlying his training prescriptions and then tailor programs to fit each athlete's specific needs and goals. Michael has coached thousands of athletes, from every major professional sport, and so what he recommends and teaches is based not on unproven hypotheses and speculation but on confirmed, time-tested outcomes.

In *New Functional Training for Sports,* Michael shares his knowledge of athlete performance development and the protocols he has refined through decades of research and experience, using thousands of clients as data points. You will find yourself soaking in a new fact or exercise technique at every turn of a page. Michael went the extra yard to educate us and equip us with the very best and most current training techniques. What he produced is an invaluable resource with benefits for both the weekend gym-goer and the seasoned strength and conditioning coach. It is my hope that you find his book as illuminating as I did.

Craig Breslow
Boston Red Sox

PREFACE

In 2002 an editor at Human Kinetics approached me to write a book on the functional training of athletes. This was a difficult task because at the time I wasn't sure I even knew what functional training was. So I asked if I could simply write what I was currently doing with my athlete clients. The editor said yes, as HK believed that the way we trained best exemplified this new concept, functional training. In my mind the way we trained was simply common sense and was founded on what I believed were the best practices at the time. Little did I know then that the book and the concepts and protocols presented in it would have such a profound effect on our field.

Additionally, to enhance *New Functional Training for Sports,* you'll get access to videos of many of the exercises presented in the book. The online video reinforces the written and pictorial instructions from the book for the exercises. Within chapters 5 through 10, you will notice a video symbol next to certain exercises. This is an indication of which exercises are included in the online video.

Much has changed since I wrote the first edition of *Functional Training for Sports.* Strength and conditioning, personal training, and physical therapy have advanced and to some degree merged into what is being labeled by some as performance development or performance enhancement. Functional training is now widely accepted as the essential way to train around the world. Big-box gyms compete for the functional training client. Every day in health clubs across the world, machines are being moved out to open up space for plyometric equipment, sleds, and kettlebells. Gyms, such as my Mike Boyle Strength and Conditioning facility near Boston, compete for members by offering not only a place to exercise but also guidance on how to train effectively and specifically in order to perform optimally and stay injury free.

Being on the forefront of the functional training revolution was gratifying professionally, but that was never my motivation. I never sought to be different or cutting edge; my sole objective was to better serve my athletes, my clients. All I've ever wanted to do was present the best program I could while allowing my athletes to excel and at the same time remain healthy.

You see, back around the turn of the century, I had become disillusioned by what I perceived to be a Faustian bargain accepted in the strength and conditioning community. Yes, we were getting athletes stronger and probably better, but at what cost? We had, as a close colleague of mine, Gray Cook, so aptly described, become very good at putting strength on top of dysfunction.

So as I considered a new edition of this book, my intent was to simply reinforce the case for functional training and update some of the exercises and equipment used—a modest effort to modernize a work that was starting to show its age. However, as I reviewed that 2004 publication, it became glaringly clear that it was not nearly as timeless as I had hoped. So much needed to be added, deleted, or changed. Central pieces of our current programming were not even mentioned in the original work. A much more extensive revision was required. Indeed, the effort became in effect a new book!

New Functional Training for Sports updates all the information contained in the original version to reflect best practices today. In addition, entire new sections were added to cover areas such as foam rolling and mobility, topics that were not mentioned in 2004. Most chapters have been completely rewritten to reflect scientific advances, philosophical changes, and additional experience gained over the last decade.

It seemed as if every time I went to simply update a chapter, I found that I needed to rewrite it. The chapter on core training (one of the longest in the book) needed to be completely updated to reflect a myriad of changes and advances in how we view core training. The chapters on lower body training also needed to be completely reworked as the line between squats and deadlifts blurred. Hex bars and kettlebells were not even a consideration in 2004, but they are now critical pieces of our lower body training philosophy. In truth, much more has changed than has stayed the same, and I am sure as you read you will see the similarity to the original work while enjoying the updates. I hope you'll also note the improved design and color-enhanced presentation of the text and photographs.

We classify our upper and lower body exercises as baseline, regressions, or progressions. Throughout the book, exercises are categorized as one of these three types. Baseline exercises are the general starting point for the average athlete. From here, the athlete either progresses or regresses. Progressions are numbered, in order from easy to difficult. Regressions are also numbered, but think easy, easier, easiest. Therefore progression 3 will be a fairly difficult exercise, while regression 3 will be very simple.

I take the role as author of this book very seriously. Having traveled around the globe since the first edition was published, I have a great appreciation of the positive impact such a resource can make, and I consider this a tremendous opportunity to educate and assist you. Therefore, my aim in *New Functional Training for Sports* is to offer a clear, accurate, and current approach to athlete performance development, founded on the best practices in functional training. And my hope is that the many recommendations, exercises, and protocols provided in the following pages will enable coaches, trainers, and athletes throughout the world to excel in their respective roles. Nothing would please me more.

Making Training More Functional

Function is, essentially, purpose. When we use the word *function* we are saying that something has a purpose. So when we apply that term to training for sports we are talking about purposeful training for sports. The idea of functional training or functional exercise actually originated in the sports medicine world. As is often the case, the thoughts and exercises used in rehab found their way from the physical therapy clinic and athletic training room into the weight room. The most basic thought was that the exercises used to return an athlete to health might also be the best exercises to maintain and improve health.

Since the concept of functional training was first applied to sports it has been misunderstood and mislabeled by many athletes and coaches. Terms such as *sport specific*, which implies that certain movements and movement patterns are specific to individual sports, have been used to describe some functional training concepts. But sport-specific training takes place with the athlete on the mat, field, or court, whereas in strength and conditioning we work to get the athlete stronger and to improve specific conditioning. Indeed, functional training may be more accurately represented by the term *sports-general training* than by the term *sport-specific training*.

Although we may deal with the smaller details of sport-specific adaptations in this book, it is important to understand that most sports possess far more similarities than differences. The sports-general school of thought views sports as being far more similar than different. Actions such as sprinting, striking, jumping, and moving laterally are general skills that apply to a broad range of sports. A sports generalist believes that speed training for all sports is similar. Fast is fast regardless of whether we are training American football players or soccer players. Core training is no different for golf than it is for hockey or tennis. In fact, speed training and core training vary very little from sport to sport.

In functional training we look at the commonalities of sport and reinforce them. At Mike Boyle Strength and Conditioning (MBSC) we have used remarkably similar programs to train Olympic gold medalists in judo and in ice hockey. In fact, if you viewed our programs, the first thing that would strike you is that no matter how different the athletes may appear the program remains similar.

THREE QUESTIONS TO DEFINE FUNCTIONAL TRAINING

To better understand the concept of functional training, ask yourself a few simple questions.

1. How many sports are played sitting down?

   As far as I can tell, only a few sports, such as rowing, are performed from a seated position. If we accept this premise, we can see that training muscles from a seated position would not be functional for most sports.

2. How many sports are played in a rigid environment where stability is provided by outside sources?

   The answer would appear to be none. Most sports are contested on fields or courts. The stability is provided by the athlete, not by some outside source. Reasoning again would tell us that most machine-based training systems are not by definition functional because the load is stabilized for the lifter by the machine. Proponents of machine-based training systems might argue that machine-based training is safer, but there is a clear trade-off for relative safety in the weight room.

   Although in theory machine-based training may result in fewer injuries during training, the lack of proprioceptive input (internal sensory feedback about position and movement) and the lack of stabilization will more than likely lead to a greater number of injuries during competition.

3. How many sports skills are performed by one joint acting in isolation?

   Again, the answer is zero. Functional training attempts to focus on multijoint movement as much as possible. Vern Gambetta and Gary Gray, two widely recognized experts on functional training, state, "Single joint movements that isolate a specific muscle are very non functional. Multi-joint movements which integrate muscle groups into movement patterns are very functional" (2002, paragraph 13).

From the answers to those three questions we could probably agree that functional training is best characterized by exercises done with the feet in contact with the ground and, with few exceptions, without the aid of machines.

Resistance to the concept of functional training often lies in the idea that "we have always done it this way." But, as Lee Cockrell appropriately asked in his book *Creating Magic*, "What if the way we have always done it was wrong?"

HOW FUNCTIONAL TRAINING WORKS

In its most basic application, a functional training program prepares an athlete to play his sport. Functional training is not about using one sport to train an athlete for another sport. That's cross-training. Many collegiate strength programs confuse the two and, as a result, train their athletes to be powerlifters and Olympic-style weightlifters as much as they do to excel in their primary sports.

Functional training on the other hand uses many concepts developed by sport coaches to train speed, strength, and power in order to improve sport performance and reduce incidence of injury. The key in taking those concepts from the track coach or powerlifting expert is to apply them intelligently to athletes. They cannot be applied blindly from one sport to another. Rather, a program should carefully blend concepts and knowledge from areas such as sports medicine, physical therapy, and sports performance to create the best possible scenario for that particular athlete.

Functional training teaches athletes how to handle their own body weight and, in that sense, somewhat resembles the calisthenics so popular in the early 20th century. The coach initially uses body weight as resistance and strives to employ positions that make sense to the participant.

Functional training intentionally incorporates balance and proprioception (body awareness) into training through the use of unilateral exercises. Gambetta and Gray (2002, paragraph 8) state, "Functional training programs need to introduce controlled amounts of instability so that the athlete must react in order to regain their own stability." The best and simplest way to introduce instability is to simply ask an athlete to perform an exercise standing on one leg. By design, functional training utilizes single-leg movements that require balance to properly develop the muscles in the way they are used in sport. Simply learning to produce force while under a heavy load and on two feet is nonfunctional for most athletes.

Functional training involves simple versions of squatting, forward bending, lunging, pushing, and pulling. The purpose is to provide a continuum of exercises that teach athletes to handle their own body weight in all planes of movement.

A final point on this: Functional training programs train *movements*, not muscles. There is no emphasis on overdeveloping strength in a particular movement; instead, emphasis is on attaining a balance between pushing and pulling strength and between knee-dominant hip extension (quadriceps and gluteals) and hip-dominant hip extension (hamstrings and gluteals).

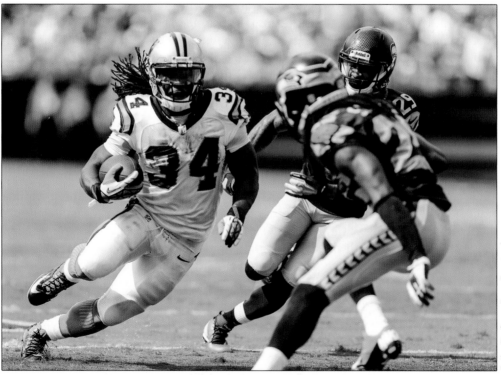

© Jim Dedmon/Icon Sportswire

Functional training helps train speed, strength, and power in order to improve sport performance and reduce incidence of injury.

The Science Behind Functional Training

To truly grasp the concept of functional training it is necessary to accept a new paradigm to explain movement. This new paradigm was first introduced by physical therapist Gary Gray in his Chain Reaction courses in the 1990s. Gray promoted a new view of muscle function based not on the old definitions of flexion, extension, adduction, and abduction but on operation of kinetic chains and the science of functional anatomy.

In the past, a version of anatomy best described as nonfunctional anatomy taught us how a muscle acted to move an isolated joint. This could also be called origin–insertion anatomy, and it worked fairly well in describing potential movement of a cadaver on a table or on a skeleton model. Origin–insertion anatomy required the memorization of where a muscle started (its origin) and ended (its insertion) and its isolated action. No thought was given to what the muscle did when a person was standing or engaged in locomotion. In contrast, functional anatomy describes how muscles act to move interrelated groups of joints and muscles working together to perform movements.

In functional anatomical terms, Gray described the actions of the lower extremity during locomotion as follows. When the foot hits the ground, every muscle from the trunk down has one simple function. The muscles of the lower body (glutes, quads, hamstrings) all act together to stop the ankle, knee, and hip from bending in order to prevent falling to the ground. In Gray's terms, all the muscles have the same function or action. The muscles all act to decelerate, or slow down, the flexion at the ankle, knee, and hip. This concept is a difficult one to accept for those who have learned conventional origin–insertion anatomy, but on further review, it makes perfect sense. In the landing phase of sprinting, is the quadriceps a knee extensor? No, when the foot hits the ground the quadriceps is actually contracting eccentrically to prevent knee flexion. Are the hamstrings a knee flexor? The hamstrings in fact are acting in a dual role to prevent both knee flexion and hip flexion.

As you think this through, the answer becomes more obvious and correspondingly easier to accept. In the landing phase of walking or running, all the muscles of the lower extremity act in concert to prevent an action, not to cause one. All the muscles eccentrically (by lengthening) decelerate, or slow down, flexion at the ankle, knee, and hip.

Once you've grasped the preceding concept, the next step comes more simply. You should now understand that after the athlete has placed the foot on the ground and decelerated flexion, all the lower-extremity muscles again act as a unit to initiate extension at the ankle, knee, and hip. In fact, the quadriceps is not just extending the knee but assisting with plantar flexion of the ankle and extension of the hip.

When viewed through the functional anatomy lens, all the muscles act eccentrically in the first sequence to stop a movement and then milliseconds later act concentrically to create a movement. If these concepts begin to make sense, you are on your way to understanding the science of functional anatomy and the concept of functional training.

When an athlete performs a nonfunctional exercise such as a leg extension, she is using a muscle action and nervous system pattern that is never employed when walking or running. The athlete is by definition performing an *open-chain* muscle action. *Open-chain* means the foot is not in contact with the ground (or a stable platform).

To exercise a muscle as it will be used, you need to close the chain and allow the muscles to work as they would when the foot is on the ground. In regard to the lower extremity, *open-chain* or *single-joint* can be considered almost synonymous with *nonfunctional*.

The Functional Training Controversy Revisited

Over the past 20 years, there has been a major shift toward attempting to make training more functional. Coaches changed from a very bilaterally based, barbell-oriented program to a program that places more emphasis on unilateral exercise and incorporates more dumbbell and kettlebell work. Gary Gray's work was the catalyst for this change.

The shift originated from the physical therapy profession, but the concept of functional training has slowly been adopted by both strength and conditioning coaches and personal trainers. It might be helpful to view strength training as a continuum, with Gray's multiplane approach on one end and the Westside Barbell powerlifting approach on the other.

The reason behind the explosive growth and rapid acceptance of functional training is simple: It makes sense to coaches and athletes and is verified from their experience in the training room and on the court, track, or field.

One of the first signs that functional training was here to stay was that the large manufacturers of the previously popular single-joint, muscle-isolating strength training machines began to introduce what they called ground-based machines and also began to manufacture basic squat racks and weight benches. The popularity of machine-based training has steadily declined as even the general public moves toward more functional training concepts.

The popularity of functional training has increased to the point that items such as foam rollers, kettlebells, and resistance bands are now available in sporting goods stores. Many health clubs have designated areas with AstroTurf and an array of functional tools for clients to practice functional training. Small-group functional training might be the largest growth area in the fitness world.

However, the initial growth period of functional training was not without controversy and detractors. This resulted from misperceptions based on lack of information and limited exposure. So, in some circles, functional training was synonymous with balance exercises and stability balls. And that view was supported, in part, by a faction of functional training proponents who wanted to accentuate the differences in their approach and deliver a clear message: Functional training should be done without machines, should be done standing, and should be multijoint. This seemed like common sense and difficult to argue with. But many coaches viewed functional training as a move away from bilateral lifting and barbells and a move toward athletes and clients lifting light weights on balance boards and balls.

Surprisingly, however, some coaches who have embraced functional training espouse concepts that, in the initial analysis, appear nonfunctional. This use of apparently nonfunctional exercises by supposed proponents of functional training caused some confusion in the field. The reasoning behind this apparent contradiction is actually simple. Function varies from joint to joint. Exercises that promote the function of joints that require stabilization are different from exercises that promote the function of joints that strive for mobility.

The primary function of certain muscles and muscle groups is stabilization. Functional training for those muscles involves training them to be better stabilizers, often by performing simple exercises through small ranges of motion. In many cases, in the effort to make everything functional, coaches and athletes ended up neglecting the important stabilizing functions of certain muscle groups.

The three key muscle groups that require stability training are the

- deep abdominals,
- hip abductors and rotators, and
- scapular stabilizers.

Many coaches began to label exercises for these areas as rehabilitative or prehabilitative, but in fact, these exercises are just another form of functional training. Function at the ankle, knee, and hip is maximized when the hip displays great stability.

For some athletes the development of stability at the hip may initially require isolated hip work to properly turn on, or activate, the muscles. Performance expert Mark Verstegen of EXOS (formerly Athletes' Performance) in Phoenix, Arizona, refers to this concept as "isolation for innervation." At certain times, certain muscle groups—notably the deep abdominals, hip abductors, and scapular stabilizers—need to be isolated to improve their function. For this reason, some apparently nonfunctional single-joint exercises may in fact improve function of the entire lower extremity. This is one of the paradoxes of functional training.

Function at the shoulder joint is enhanced by improving the function of the scapular stabilizers and rotator cuff. Although many athletes perform exercises for the rotator cuff, few exercise scapular stabilizers. But performing sports skills without strong scapular stabilizers is like trying to shoot a cannon from a canoe. At our training facility, most athletes have both inadequate rotator cuff strength and insufficient strength or control of the scapular stabilizers. As a result, we frequently employ exercises to work on the scapular stabilizers and rotator cuff that might appear nonfunctional, but the development of these areas is critical for long-term health of the shoulder joint.

Physical therapists are again leading the way in developing the stabilizers of the lower back. Improving abdominal strength to aid in the stabilization of the lower back is far from a new concept, but the specific methods are changing rapidly.

The key to developing a truly functional training program is not to go too far in any particular direction. The majority of exercises should be done standing and should be multijoint, but at the same time, attention should be paid to development of the key stabilizer groups in the hips, core, and posterior shoulder.

A second functional paradox revolves around multiplanar activity done in a sport-specific position. Advocates of this style of functional training espouse loaded exercises (i.e., done with a dumbbell or weight vest) in a flexed posture and using foot positions that some strength and conditioning coaches would consider less than desirable.

Although athletes find themselves in compromised positions in competitive situations, coaches need to evaluate how far they are willing to go in loading athletes in positions of spinal flexion. As an example, although a baseball player often squats down to field a ground ball with a flexed spine, weighted squatting movements with the spine in a flexed position may not be wise. At what point do you cross the line from safe training into unsafe training? Our position on this is simple. The argument that "this happens in sports all the time" is not sufficient to take risks in the weight room. When training for strength, never compromise back safety to make the body position of the exercise more specific.

As you begin to explore the concept of functional training for sport, keep an open mind about how and why athletes move in your sport. Think of your training as a vehicle to improve performance, not just to improve strength. Many athletes have neglected strength training because they do not fully understand the performance-enhancing value of strength in sports such as baseball, tennis, or soccer. The key from the athlete's standpoint is for the training to make sense. The key from the coach's standpoint is to make the training make sense to the athlete. A training

A CASE FOR SPORTS-GENERAL TRAINING

Olympic gold medalist Kayla Harrison is a great example of how sports-general training can benefit an athlete. In Kayla's program we did not need to imitate the throws of judo; we simply needed to get her stronger in basic movement patterns. The important thing for Kayla was to develop strength in pushing, pulling, rotating, squatting, and lunging. How we chose to do that was based not on sport but on injury history and sport demands.

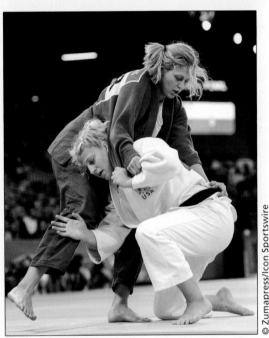

© Zumapress/Icon Sportswire

Judo demands a high amount of practice time and a lot of high-impact body stress. We chose brief twice-weekly workouts focusing on the basic push, pull, knee dominant, hip dominant, core theme, to be repeated over and over.

Because judo is a year-round sport, the program was a version of the basic two-day programs you will see in the last chapter. There was very little attempt to imitate judo and a strong emphasis on the basics of strength and conditioning as we see them.

A typical training day for Kayla consisted of the following:

Foam roller

Stretching

Dynamic warm-up

Power: medicine ball drills and plyometrics

Strength: push (dumbbell bench press), pull (ring row), knee dominant (single-leg squat), and hip dominant (single-leg straight-leg deadlift)

Core: done between sets (basic exercises such as plank, side plank, and carries)

Conditioning: specific four-minute bouts that match the energy demands of judo, done primarily on a stationary bike to save joint stress program built around actions that do not occur in sport simply does not make sense. The key is to design programs that truly prepare athletes for their sports. This can be done only by using exercises that train the muscles the same way they are used in sport—in other words, through functional training.

For the strength and conditioning professional, the number one goal of a strength and conditioning program should be injury reduction. In professional sports, the success or failure of the strength and conditioning program is measured by player health more than by wins and losses. NFL football uses a stat called starters games missed, baseball monitors days on the disabled list, and hockey looks at man games lost to injury. In each case player health seems to correlate with sound strength and conditioning programs and team success. On the flip side, if coaches employ a system of training that results in few training injuries but does not reduce competitive injuries, are they doing their job or protecting their job?

The key to every functional program is this: Practice what you preach and keep it simple.

REFERENCES

Cockrell, L. 2008. *Creating Magic.* Crown Business.

Gambetta, V., and G. Gray. 2002. *The Gambetta Method: Common Sense Guide to Training for Functional Performance.* Gambetta Sports Training Systems: Sarasota, FL.

CHAPTER 2

Analyzing the Demands of the Sport

Before you can design an effective functional training program, you must first analyze and understand the demands of the sport. Think about the sport. See a picture in your mind. What type of sport is it?

Most sports are either endurance sports or speed and power sports. Almost all team sports are speed and power sports. Individual sports such as gymnastics and figure skating also rely primarily on speed and power. Racket sports, including tennis, are speed and power sports.

Now ask yourself who the dominant players or performers are in the sport. Are they the athletes with the best endurance or the best flexibility? Most often neither is the case. Usually the best players or top performers are the most efficient and explosive movers. Speed and agility are the most prized qualities in almost every fast-paced power sport.

MATCHING TYPE OF SPORT AND TYPE OF TESTS

Back in the early 1980s, when professional sports teams and top amateur and professional athletes began to seek training advice, they often turned to the wrong people. Consultants employed by professional teams and sport federations were most often exercise physiologists with little or no experience in addressing the needs of athletes in speed and power sports. Generally, they were endurance-sport athletes themselves.

So, rather than evaluating and prescribing in a manner most suited to speed and power sports, the exercise physiologists applied the same generic protocol as they did for all athletes:

1. Test the athletes.

2. Analyze the tests.

3. Draw conclusions.

Unfortunately, this very simple method for attempting to improve athletes' fitness and performance was filled with flaws, many of which continue to plague strength and conditioning professionals three decades later.

Most speed and power athletes perform poorly on tests of steady-state aerobic capacity ($\dot{V}O_2$). For simplicity's sake, such tests are generally performed on cycle ergometers, but these athletes do not regularly train on a bike. The conclusion, based on $\dot{V}O_2$ scores, was that the athletes were unfit. The plan to make them fit almost always emphasized the improvement of the athletes' aerobic capacity. The rationale was that a player with a higher maximal oxygen uptake would be able to play longer and recover more rapidly. All of this seemed scientific and valid. However, there are a number of reasons why this approach does not meet the needs of athletes in speed and power sports:

- Athletes in sports that use primarily fast-twitch muscles and explosive movements generally perform poorly on tests of aerobic capacity. This is not a new discovery.

- Well-conditioned athletes in sports of an intermittent nature (i.e., most team sports) may not necessarily perform well in steady-state tests of aerobic capacity, particularly when the test is done on an apparatus (such as a bike) that is not the athletes' primary mode of training.

- Steady-state or long-distance training to improve the fitness or aerobic capacity of fast and explosive athletes often detracts from the physiological qualities that make these athletes special.

- Explosive athletes frequently develop overuse injuries when required to perform extensive amounts of steady-state work.

- The technology used to improve aerobic capacity may in fact be the enemy. Lack of ground contact and lack of hip extension can set an athlete up for numerous injuries.

Cyclists should ride bikes, rowers should row, athletes who have to run fast should run fast on the ground, and athletes who have to jump should jump. Cross-training may be a good idea in limited volumes but should be used as an active rest or injury-avoidance tool. Too much dependence on any technology can have a price.

We can now, many years later, see clearly that exercise physiologists looked at the problem of improving athletes' fitness and performance from the wrong perspective. You don't simply analyze a top performer and seek to improve his weakness. By blindly attempting to improve what is perceived as a weakness, a coach in fact may be detracting from a strength. This is particularly applicable when training young people. When coaching young athletes, emphasis should be placed on the development of qualities such as speed and power over the development of general fitness.

TRAIN SLOW, PLAY SLOW

Many an athlete has performed poorly because of a simple training mistake: cross country. Countless athletes (often escorted by their upset parents) have come to me after a disappointing season for which they believed they had trained so hard. They can't figure out why all those miles they ran never paid off. Some even report feeling a step slow, lacking that burst—quick, explosive movement—when they needed it.

And it is all I can do not to ask: Are you really surprised? Instead, I point out some facts. No team sports entails running for miles at a time. Even if you do run miles in a game, as in soccer, those miles are a series of sprints interspersed with a series of walks or jogs. In hockey the athletes perform a short series of sprints, sit down a few minutes, and then repeat. Running long distances does not prepare an athlete to run short distances, and certainly not to sprint repeatedly.

There is a concept called sport-specific training. As the phrase suggests, it holds that the best way to condition for a sport is to mimic the energy systems demanded in playing that sport. If the sport is sprint, jog, walk, then the training is sprint, jog, walk. Makes perfect sense.

There is another very important concept to grasp here: Train slow, get slow. The reality is it is very difficult to make someone fast and very easy to make someone slow. If you want to get an athlete slow, simply ask her to run slower, longer. Simple. She may be in shape, but it is the wrong shape.

Another problem with a steady-state sport such as cross country is injuries. Something like 60 percent of the people who take up running get injured. Those are lousy odds if you're looking to be healthy to start a season.

Athletes who dominate their sports are those who run the fastest, jump the highest, and have the quickest burst. Yes, conditioning matters, but train for the sport. Lift weights, jump, sprint. The key is to gain strength and power in the off-season.

Simply put, an athlete who is not a cross country runner shouldn't run cross country. Athletes who want to get faster and get in great sport condition need to train the way the best athletes train—using a combination of strength training and interval training to prepare properly.

IDENTIFYING AND IMPROVING KEY QUALITIES

Noted speed expert Charlie Francis wrote a landmark work in 1986 called *The Charlie Francis Training System* (reissued as *Training for Speed*, Francis 1997). In it he described the characteristics of a sprinter and how to properly train these characteristics. This information has been the basis for our program design and philosophy since that time.

Francis coached many top sprinters, including record-setting sprinter Ben Johnson. And, although tainted a bit by Johnson's use of anabolic steroids, Francis' accomplishments as a coach cannot be overstated. Canada was not considered a hotbed of sprinting, but Francis developed world record holders in a country without a huge population base. His athletes won gold medals at the Olympic Games, world championships, and Commonwealth Games.

Francis came to simple and logical conclusions about developing sprinters. He believed there must be sufficient power-related training during an athlete's early years (ages 13 to 17) to maintain the genetically determined level of white (fast-twitch or power-related) muscle fiber. Power-related work also promotes the shift of transitional fiber to power-related muscle fiber. Francis (1997) states, "Endurance work must be carefully limited to light-light/medium volumes to prevent the conversion of transitional or intermediate muscle fiber to red, endurance muscle fiber."

Francis believed not only that can you make an athlete into a sprinter but also, more importantly, that you might negatively affect an athlete's ability to develop speed by focusing on endurance. In other words, it's easy to make a sprinter into an endurance athlete, but this is seldom a desirable result.

The bigger and more important point here is that it is essential to analyze a sport to ascertain the qualities that make a great performer and then to develop a program to improve those qualities. That is much different from analyzing a performer and trying to improve what he does not do well.

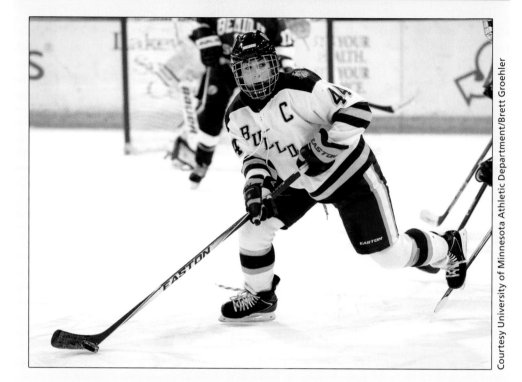

Courtesy University of Minnesota Athletic Department/Brett Groehler

Zoe Hickel was captain of the University of Minnesota Duluth's women's hockey team. She was a perfect example of an athlete who worked hard and was in great condition but was probably emphasizing the wrong qualities. As an 18-year-old Zoe was one of the top collegiate recruits and had represented the United States on the women's national under-18 team. However, three years of hard work in college had actually managed to decrease her vertical jump and probably limit her effectiveness.

In 2014 Zoe moved to Boston for an internship at Mike Boyle Strength and Conditioning and focused on our program, which features little to no endurance training and no long, slow distance work. Zoe's longest run of the summer was probably a 300-yard shuttle run.

In just seven weeks Zoe increased her vertical jump by three inches (back to her level of three years earlier), gained six pounds, and was now properly prepared for her first national tryout camp in four years. The keys were a significant decrease in endurance work, an increased emphasis on lower body strength, and a program designed to gain lean mass. Zoe was the leading scorer in camp and earned a spot on the U.S. women's national team. Not surprisingly, Hickel also had her best offensive year, leading UMD in scoring with 19 goals and 13 assists and earning All-League honors.

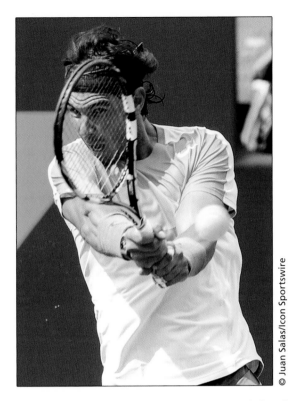

© Juan Salas/Icon Sportswire

To train for sports such as tennis, athletes must sprint and decelerate, not just do 5-mile runs.

For years coaches have been trying to improve the aerobic capacity of explosive athletes. The end result seems to be an athlete with a higher oxygen uptake but no real change in performance. Training programs designed in this way improve the athlete's ability to work at a sustained pace in sports that do not require a sustained pace.

The defenders of this practice point to the importance of the aerobic system to recovery and tell us things like "A soccer player runs five miles in a soccer match" or "A tennis match can last two hours." This point is not contestable. The question is, At what speed and in what time period? A tennis match may take two hours to play, but what is the ratio of sprinting to standing? Are the players in constant motion? The advocates of aerobic training never point to this training as a way to improve performance, only as a way to improve recovery. The goal is to improve performance.

A soccer match is actually a series of sprints, jogs, and walks that occur over two hours. Any athlete can run five miles in two hours. In fact, five miles in two hours is two point five miles per hour. That is a slow walk pace. Most unfit people can walk five miles in two hours. The important point is that great soccer players can accelerate and decelerate repeatedly during these two hours. Now ask yourself, "How does an athlete condition for soccer?"

To train for sports such as soccer or tennis, athletes must sprint and decelerate, often from top speed, to be prepared to play the game. Will they develop this ability in five-mile runs? Probably not. The same logic can apply to almost any power sport. In football the athlete generally runs 10 yards or less. The plays take 5 seconds. There is almost 40 seconds of rest between plays. How should you condition for football? Probably with short sprints with 30- to 40-second rests. This is the key to analyzing a sport. Watch the game. Watch the great players. Look for the common denominators. Don't focus on what they can't do; try to figure out why the great athletes do things well. Don't continue to accept what is viewed as common knowledge if it defies common sense.

To analyze a sport ask yourself a few questions:

- Does the sport require sprinting or jumping? If so, then lower body strength (particularly the single-leg variety) is critical.
- Are you required to stop and start frequently in your sport?
- How long is the event, or how long does a play last? (This is a bit complicated, but think about the total length of a game, program, or routine; or think about how long the rest is between shifts, plays, or points.)
- Are the players on the field, ice, track, or court the entire time?
- If yes, how often do they sprint, and how often do they jog? Do they jog for extended periods of time (more than five minutes)? If not, then why do it in training?
- Does an athlete's speed and power place her in the top 10 percent of athletes in her sport? [Male athletes: Can I complete the 10-yard dash in under 1.65 electronic? (*Electronic* refers to more accurate electronic timing rather than a handheld stopwatch.) Can I jump vertically over 34 inches (86 cm)? Female athletes: Can I complete the 10-yard dash in under 1.85 electronic? Can I jump vertically over 25 inches (64 cm)? If the answers are no, you can always use more speed and power.]

Speed and power are essential for almost all sports. Tennis, soccer, baseball, gymnastics, figure skating, and other sports too numerous to mention all rely heavily on power and speed. The key to improving sport performance lies in improving the ability to produce speed and power. Endurance should be an afterthought. We tell our athletes over and over that it takes years to get fast and powerful and mere weeks to get in aerobic shape. With this in mind as you continue to read, think about how you are currently training yourself or your athletes and how you might train smarter.

REFERENCES

Francis, C. 1997. *Training for Speed*. Ottawa, Ontario: TBLI Publications.

CHAPTER 3

Assessing Functional Strength

As stated in chapter 1, functional training is training that makes sense. After analyzing the demands of the sport, the next step is to gauge your strengths and weaknesses or the strengths and weaknesses of your athletes. The tests in this chapter allow for self-assessment.

It is extremely rare to find an athlete who has too much strength, too much power, or too much speed for his sport. You rarely hear a television commentator say, "Boy, he was so fast he ran right by that ball." Think of strength as the road to speed and power. The key is to develop functional strength, strength an athlete can use.

Objective measurement of functional strength can be humbling for even the best athletes. To assess functional strength, athletes must move against a resistance in a manner that is likely to occur in sport or life. So it makes sense that one's own body weight—the most common form of resistance—is most frequently employed in functional strength assessment exercises.

A typical strength test requires the athlete to move a predetermined amount of weight in an exercise for which there are readily available norms. For example, the bench press is a test frequently used to measure upper body strength. But does such a test tell us much about an athlete's functional strength?

Remember too that raw numbers must be put into context. In most cases an athlete who can bench-press 350 pounds (160 kg) would be considered strong. But what if the athlete weighs 350 pounds? The athlete can then bench-press only his own body weight. Don't be fooled by the number; athletes need to perform functional exercises with their body weight.

Those who advocate the development of functional strength question the value of a test in which the athlete lies on the back. In most sports, lying on the back indicates a failure to perform at a high level. We tell our football players this: If you are lying on your back pushing up, you stink at football. Does this mean you cannot bench-press in a functional program? No, you can use the bench press to develop general upper body strength, but if you cannot perform body-weight exercises such as push-ups and chin-ups, then you are not functionally strong and may be more likely to be injured.

A good functional strength training program employs both tried and true strength exercises such as the bench press and less conventional exercises such as a single-leg squat, a rear-foot-elevated split squat, a push-up, or a single-leg straight-leg deadlift. The key is to make the program more functional without throwing out the baby with the bathwater. Methods that have been used to develop strength successfully for 50 years need not always be sacrificed just to have a more functional program.

On the other side of the coin, don't just develop strength for strength's sake. For too long we have relied on sports such as powerlifting or Olympic weightlifting to define our athletes' strength levels. Coaches often have imitated or copied other sports in their attempts to make their athletes better. The key in functional training is to develop usable strength.

However, functional training does not need to be an either/or proposition. Too often in the field of strength and conditioning, coaches attempt to adhere to one school of thought as opposed to developing appropriate training programs for their athletes. Athletes in training are not necessarily powerlifters or Olympic lifters, so the objective should be to combine knowledge from a number of disciplines to provide the best training program possible. In the words of EXOS performance coach Denis Logan, we need to "develop great athletes that are good weightlifters."

ASSESSING FUNCTIONAL UPPER BODY STRENGTH

So, how best to determine an athlete's functional strength? Over the years I've found three simple tests to be most effective and accurate in the assessment of functional upper body strength.

Maximum Number of Chin-Ups or Pull-Ups

Correct chin-up (palms toward the face) and pull-up (palms away from face) technique is essential for accurate assessment. Elbows must be extended after each rep is completed, and the shoulder blades must abduct to produce visible movement (see figure 3.1). Don't count any reps not done to full extension or any reps in which the chin does not get above the bar.

Kipping (using momentum to move the body) is not allowed. Most athletes who claim they can do large numbers of pull-ups or chin-ups actually perform half or three-quarter reps.

Athletes who cannot do a chin-up are not functionally strong and may be more likely to be injured, particularly in the shoulder. Most athletes will take up to one year to achieve even the high school level if they have not regularly performed chin-ups.

In order to improve at chin-ups, an athlete cannot follow a program of pull-down exercises. Instead, exercises such as assisted chin-ups and or chin-ups with an eccentric emphasis (10- to 20-second lowerings from the bar) must be done. Please refer to chapter 8 for detailed chin-up progressions.

We have adapted our standards and now require athletes to move to a weighted chin-up once they can do 10 chin-ups. Once an athlete does 10 reps at body weight, he is required to add a 25-pound (10 kg) weight suspended from a dip belt for the next test. Generally this brings the reps down from 10 to 3, but most importantly it forces the athlete to strength-train. As strength is the goal, we want the test to reinforce our path toward the goal.

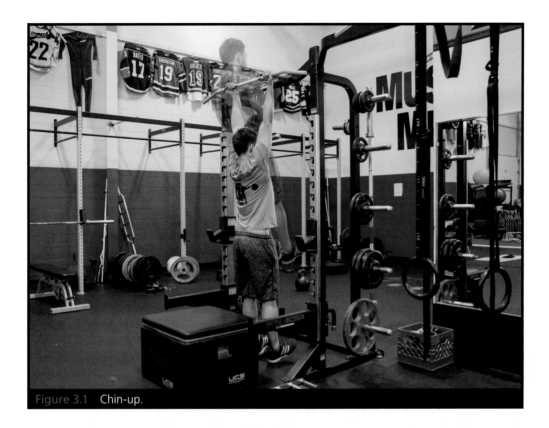

Figure 3.1 Chin-up.

The maximum number of chin-ups or pull-ups may be used to determine the weights used for weighted repetitions. Using this type of testing and training progression, we now have female athletes who can perform five reps with 45 pounds (20 kg) and male athletes who use over 90 pounds (40 kg) for weighted chin-ups.

Maximum Number of Suspension Inverted Rows

The suspension inverted row is the reverse of the bench press and primarily works the scapular retractors, shoulder muscles involved in pulling movements. If athletes cannot perform a suspension inverted row, they lack upper back strength and should begin with the basic rowing progressions described in chapter 8. An athlete who lacks upper back strength is at greater risk for problems related to the shoulder's rotator cuff. This is of particular importance to athletes prone to rotator cuff problems such as swimmers, tennis players, pitchers, quarterbacks, and other throwing athletes.

The athlete places the feet on a bench or plyo box and grips the handles or rings as if to perform a bench press. The suspension apparatus should be set at about waist height. With the entire body held rigid, the athlete pulls the handles to the chest. The thumbs must touch the chest, with no change in body position. Make sure there is full extension of the elbow and the body is kept perfectly straight. Count only the reps in which the thumbs touch the body while the body remains straight (see figure 3.2).

As with the chin-up, once an athlete can perform 10 reps a 10-pound (5 kg) weight vest is added. Again, the focus is on the development of strength, not endurance.

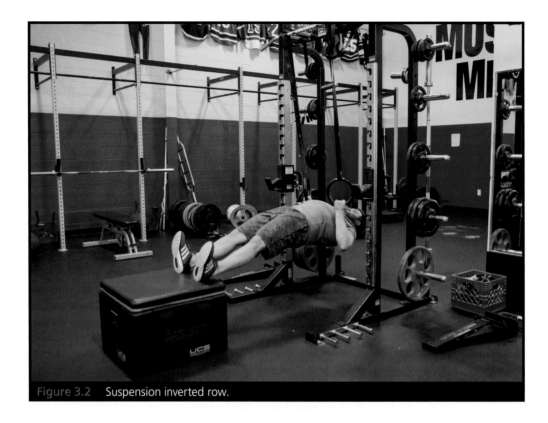

Figure 3.2   Suspension inverted row.

Maximum Number of Push-Ups

This is a much more accurate test for larger athletes than the bench press. For each push-up, the chest should touch a two-inch-thick (5 cm) foam pad and the torso should stay rigid. The head must stay in line with the torso. Do not count reps in which back position is not maintained, the chest does not touch the pad, the head protrudes, or the elbows are not fully extended. To prevent cheating and make counting simple, use a metronome set at 50 beats per minute. The athlete should keep pace with the metronome, going up on the first beat and down on the next. The test is over when the athlete fails to do another push-up or cannot keep pace with the metronome.

As in the previous two tests, once the athlete completes 10 reps, a weighted vest (initially a 10-pound [5 kg] vest and then a 20-pound [10 kg] vest) is added. For further progression, higher reps can be done once the 20-pound vest is used, or plates can be placed on the back.

ASSESSING FUNCTIONAL LOWER BODY STRENGTH

Safely and accurately assessing functional lower body strength is significantly more difficult than assessing upper body strength. In fact, few reliable tests exist that safely measure functional lower body strength. The conventional double-leg back squat has been used for many years to test lower body strength, but the safety of that test is questionable, particularly when done for one maximum repetition. In addition, many practitioners view the back squat as an exercise adopted from training for American football, and thus not suitable for the needs in their sport.

Rear-Foot-Elevated Split Squat

Over the past five years we have attempted to develop and administer a valid, reliable, and safe lower body test that is also simple to perform. We have begun using maximum reps, or RM (most repetitions an athlete can perform at a prese-lected load), of the rear-foot-elevated split squat as a test of functional lower body strength. Although it's not perfect, we've found the test to be effective both in assessing strength and gauging progress.

The test is relatively simple. The athlete places the back foot on a conventional exercise bench or a specially designed stand, with an Airex pad on the floor to protect the knee from the repeated contact. The athlete selects a load in the 5RM range and then performs as many repetitions as possible until technical failure (i.e., until she can no longer maintain perfect technique).

Loads typically entail two dumbbells or two kettlebells. Kettlebells are preferred because they are easier to hold. This side loading is preferred to a back or front squat position for safety reasons. Failure with dumbbells held at the sides will simply result in a pair of dumbbells on the floor. Failure in a back or front squat position could result in unsafe, compromising positions.

Another possibility is to test single-leg squats. We have found that functionally strong athletes can perform sets of five single-leg squats while holding 5-pound (2.5 kg) dumbbells by the beginning of the fourth week of a properly designed training program (see figure 3.3). Athletes unfamiliar with or unaccustomed to single-leg strength work should progress through three weeks of split squats (both feet on the floor) or three weeks of rear-foot-elevated split squats (back foot elevated) before beginning single-leg squats. Our elite females can do 10 repetitions with 40 pounds (20 kg) of total weight (20-pound vest and 10-pound dumbbells), while our males can handle up to 100 pounds (45 kg) of total external load. Weighted repetitions can get difficult for males because multiple layers of weight vests are needed.

Finally, it is nearly impossible to safely assess functional lower body strength without first teaching the athlete the exercise used in the test. If this is not possible, then the risk far outweighs the potential benefits of any information obtained.

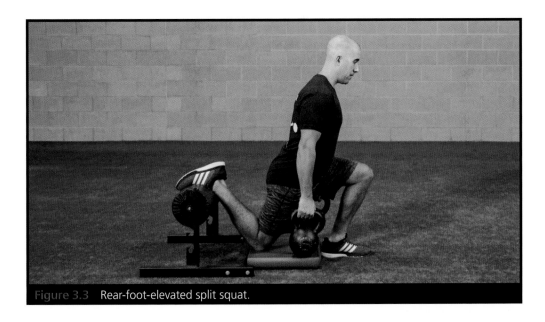

Figure 3.3   Rear-foot-elevated split squat.

Double-Leg Vertical Jump

A simple alternative is to use the double-leg vertical jump (see figure 3.4) to assess leg power and then to reassess leg power after a proper strength program has been initiated. The vertical jump test is relatively safe to administer and has readily available norms. Increases in leg power will be at least partially attributable to increases in leg strength.

The Just Jump System and Vertec are the best devices for evaluating the vertical jump, although both methods have inherent flaws. (Both devices are distributed by M-F Athletic Company and can be purchased at www.performbetter.com.)

Just Jump is a device that measures time in the air and converts it to inches. The athlete must jump and land in the same place, and the athlete must land toes first with no knee lift or knee bend. All these factors may influence the score.

Vertec is an adjustable device that measures both reach height and jump height. With Vertec, the reach measurement must be accurate. At our training facility, we test a two-hand reach and a one-hand touch on the jump. Consistency among testers and in test administration is essential.

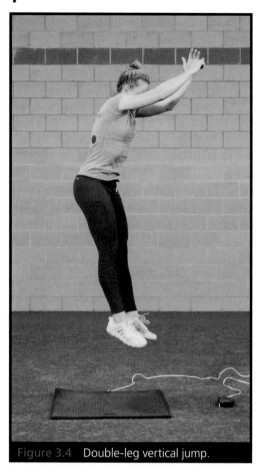

Figure 3.4   Double-leg vertical jump.

CLOSING POINTS ON FUNCTIONAL STRENGTH TESTING

Tests are used to evaluate progress. They are not the program and should not be the program. Testing only shows what areas are in need of training and what areas may be prone to injury. But the numbers obtained from testing are helpful in motivating and monitoring subsequent strength development.

Some coaches may criticize the testing protocols presented in this chapter because some of the tests can be construed as tests of muscular endurance, even though the number of repetitions are capped. Although I somewhat agree, it must be stated again that the tests are not the training program, only a method of evaluating progress.

At this point you should better understand the demands of the sport and have an idea of your strength level or the strength level of your athletes. Hopefully, the principles of functional training are becoming clearer to you. The idea is to develop a plan that makes sense for the sport and strengthens areas that are key to performance or to injury prevention. The evaluation of functional strength is an important step in developing a training plan to improve. The next step is to develop the plan.

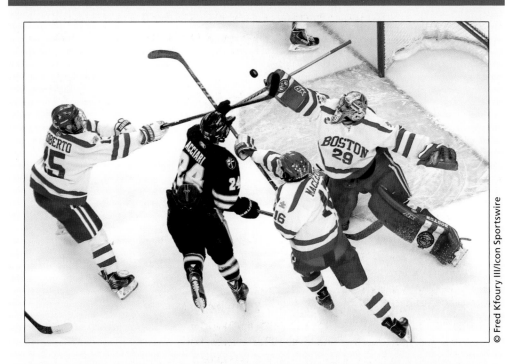

© Fred Kfoury III/Icon Sportswire

We instituted a battery of functional strength tests similar to those described in this chapter with the Boston University men's hockey team, and the results in terms of strength gain and injury prevention were outstanding. Our average 1RM in the chin-up was 100 pounds (45 kg) when we tested.

Initially, 10 to 15 body-weight chin-ups was considered an excellent performance; five years later it would be considered below average. In our gym it is normal to see everyone performing weighted chin-ups, and it is not unusual to see males performing reps with 45-pound (20 kg) plates.

It is also worth noting that we had very few collision-related shoulder injuries on our BU teams. This is strong evidence for the injury prevention benefits of a balance of pushing and pulling movements against resistance in training.

Designing a Program

I talk frequently with coaches about sport performance programming. Often the conversation starts something like this: "I use a little of your stuff, a little of Mark Verstegen's stuff, and mix in a little of . . ." This is almost always meant as a compliment, but it comes off a different way.

When it comes to developing new performance programs or adopting all or parts of existing programs, an analogy from the culinary industry applies. Some people can really cook; others need cookbooks and recipes. Some people write cookbooks; others read cookbooks. Even in the restaurant world, there are cooks and there are chefs. Cooks follow the recipes, while chefs create the recipes.

So are you a cook or a chef? If you are creating your first program for yourself or for a team, you are a cook. Find a good recipe that meets your needs and follow it exactly. Furthermore, in cooking, every ingredient in a recipe has a purpose. Most baked foods require flour, for example. You wouldn't bake a cake and leave out the flour, would you?

If you were cooking something for the first time, would you take two recipes from two different cookbooks and combine them? Would you add ingredients from one of the recipes while subtracting ingredients from the other? If you did this, would the end product be good? No. The same thing happens when coaches develop their performance training programs from a mixture of sources.

Unfortunately, when it comes to program design, this is exactly what many coaches do. I have athletes who have trained with me for years and eventually become coaches themselves. Instead of using the program that was so successful for them, they alter it. Then they email me the program and say, "Can you look this over?" Invariably the program is a little of mine and a little of theirs, with maybe a touch of a third party's. A combination of recipes if you will. Also, invariably the program is poor. These are not experienced "chefs," yet they have chosen to alter the recipe to suit their taste. The better choice is to choose a recipe created by an experienced chef and then do a great job of making the meal. In other words, coach the heck out of the program.

If you have been developing programs for a few years, your expertise might be the equivalent of a sous-chef's. The sous-chef is the second in command in the kitchen. Many third- and fourth-year coaches are sous-chefs. They have developed the ability to alter the recipe without spoiling the meal. They understand that ingredients can be altered but that there should be a plan. They also understand that the plan should be followed. The sous-chef knows that the ratio of ingredients matters and that you don't simply cook to your own taste.

Finally, after five years of successful program design, you might qualify as a chef. At this point you can contemplate bold changes to the recipe because you have extensive experience cooking and baking. One noted strength and conditioning coach used to say, "It's okay to break the rules. Just make sure you understand the rules first." After five years you should not be looking at new training DVDs and scrapping your whole program. Chefs don't abandon their chosen cooking approach in favor of the latest trend. Instead, you make minor adjustments that you believe will further refine your system.

My experience suggests that most coaches need more direction in performance training program design. Don't be afraid to copy if you are a beginner. In fact, I would encourage you to copy rather than to mix. The programs in this book are provided for just that purpose. I would rather you copy my program than attempt to add bits of the recipe in this book to the recipes of others.

In previous writings I have warned that it is a mistake to simply copy programs. What I should have said is that it is a mistake to *blindly* copy programs. So be informed, and be careful and discerning in your choice. But if you are not confident or prepared to create a program, feel free to copy. Cookbooks were created for a reason.

PROGRAM BASICS

Once you have honestly assessed where you fit on the program design proficiency continuum, the next step is to ensure you understand the underlying concepts. This chapter will familiarize you with the concepts of program design, the tools used to implement those concepts, and how to properly progress a functional training program.

Programming for Conditioning and Fitness

Every program must start with a two- or three-week base-building period. For athletes in great shape already, this preparatory period keeps their fitness from declining. For athletes with any significant deficit in their baseline fitness, it will sound an alarm.

The preparatory period should consist of tempo running to develop a base of sprint-related conditioning. Tempo running is neither sprinting nor jogging. It consists of runs of various distances (generally 100 or 200 yards or meters) interspersed with walking recovery. At our training facility, athletes frequently stride the length of our 40-yard turf, turn, and stride back. A stride is in that middle ground between a jog and a sprint. We also do tempo runs on our treadmills, picking a moderate stride pace (9 to 10 MPH), and do intervals such as 15 on, 30 off or 20 on, 40 off.

After ensuring an adequate fitness base you can start designing a functional exercise program. The emphasis is not just on improving strength but also on creating strength that can be used in sport or in life.

To begin, review these basic questions posed in chapter 2:

- Is your sport a sprint-dominated sport that emphasizes speed and power?
- Are you required to stop and start frequently in your sport?
- How long does a play, point, shift, or routine last in your sport?

After analyzing what actually happens in a game, choose conditioning activities that attempt to mimic the energy systems and style of the game. Then be specific: Athletes need to be told how far to run, how fast to run, and how much rest to take between runs. Athletes allowed to run at their own pace usually run too slowly. Athletes allowed to control their own rest periods most often rest too long.

Soccer, field hockey, lacrosse, basketball, and ice hockey, for example, are all sprint-dominated sports in which athletes stop and start frequently. It makes sense, then, that training should feature stop-and-start conditioning activities, such as the 300-yard shuttle run.

Programming for Strength

From a strength standpoint, most sports are the same. One of my favorite quotes was provided by Marco Cardinale, high-performance director for London 2012, at a seminar I attended in Boston. "Your sport is not different, you just think it is."

Cardinale was referring to his experiences trying to coordinate strength and conditioning for the London Olympics. All the coaches believed their programs needed to be different because their sport was unique. The truth is that the basic strength training needs are pretty much alike across sports. And, even if they were different, it would not drastically change the way you strength-train. The conditioning aspect of practice might be different, but strength training probably follows the 80–20 rule, or the Pareto principle. Eighty percent of what we do in the weight room will be the same for every sport. Every athlete has the same sets of muscles, and strengthening those muscles will be amazingly similar.

Strength is needed to facilitate power and speed. Think of strength as the base on which everything else is built. However, don't think of the simple concept of bilateral strength; rather, focus on specific unilateral strength.

A strength program is as simple as a push, a pull, a knee-dominant exercise, a hip-dominant exercise, and some core work. I have had the pleasure of coaching or training Olympic medalists and world champions in basketball, football, ice hockey, soccer, judo, rowing, and a host of other sports. I can tell you that 80–20 is accurate, and if it is not, it's closer to 90–10 than 70–30.

ESSENTIALS OF PROGRAM DESIGN

To properly design a functional strength training program, keep the following principles in mind.

■ *Learn the basic patterns first.* Master the movement basics before considering progressions to make an exercise program more functional. The biggest mistake is for athletes who are not competent in a basic movement, such as the squat, to attempt to load or advance the movement. An athlete must first master the body-weight versions of every exercise before loading the exercises. Then and only then should you follow the recommended progressions.

■ *Begin with simple body-weight exercises.* The number one way to destroy a strength program is by attempting to lift too much weight too soon. If an athlete can perform an exercise with body weight but struggles with an external load, then obviously the external load is the problem. Either reduce or eliminate the external load. For upper body pulling or rowing movements, many athletes are unable to begin with even body-weight resistance. In this case, machines or elastic assistance may be necessary.

■ *Progress from simple to complex.* The progressions in this book were developed over many years. Follow the progressions. For single-leg exercises, the athlete should master the simplest exercise, such as the split squat, before progressing to a more complex exercise such as the rear-foot-elevated split squat. The exercises follow a functional progression and add increasing levels of difficulty at the appropriate time as needed.

■ *Use the concept of progressive resistance.* Progressive resistance is the key to success. In the simplest sense, try to add weight or reps every week. If an athlete does the same weight for one or two more reps, she has made progress. If an athlete uses a weight that is 5 pounds (2.5 kg) heavier for the same number of reps, he has made progress. We have built Olympic and world champions with these simple principles. Progressive resistance is credited to Milo of Crete, who eventually carried a bull by beginning with a calf and carrying it every day as it grew. As the calf grew to a bull, Milo's strength grew with it. This is the simple basis for strength training.

For body-weight exercise, the progression is simple. Begin with three sets of 8 repetitions in week 1, move to three sets of 10 in week 2, and finish with three sets of 12 in week 3. This is simple progressive resistance training utilizing just body weight.

By the fourth week, you can generally progress to a more difficult exercise or add external loads. External resistance can be a dumbbell, a kettlebell, a weight vest, a sandbag, or a medicine ball. These more difficult exercises can then be progressed by the same method (8-10-12) or through basic resistance concepts. Simply adding 5 pounds per week to an exercise can theoretically result in an increase of 260 pounds (120 kg) per year. Most athletes dream about gains like this, and in reality, most athletes eventually plateau on this type of program, but beginners can progress for a long time with basic resistance progression.

One word of advice in program design: Don't design a program based on what you like or dislike as a coach or trainer; design a program that works for the athlete.

Periodization

Periodization might be the most overstudied subject in the training world. Tens of thousands of pages have been written detailing the complexities of microcycles and mesocycles. And this has only served to confuse what should be a fairly simple concept, as articulated by strength and conditioning legend Charles Poliquin in the 1988 article "Variety in Strength Training": "Phases of high volume (accumulation, extensive loading), high intensity (intensification, intensive loading) and unloading should be modulated within the program."

It really is that simple. Higher-volume, lower-load periods should be alternated with higher-intensity, lower-volume periods. Dan John, another giant in the field, recommended between 15 and 25 reps for major exercises. That means you have the choice of accumulating volume with three sets of eight (24 reps) or exercising more intensely with three sets of five (15 reps).

The big takeaway is to write simple programs and coach them. A well-coached bad program will beat a poorly coached good program every time. The devil is in the details of the execution.

PROGRESSIVE RESISTANCE TRAINING AND BASIC PERIODIZATION

Our program is a simple periodization cycle of sets of 8 to 10 (accumulation), followed by sets of three (intensification) and then sets of five. There is nothing fancy about what we do, but we do strive to add weight or reps every week. Our athletes have used these techniques to develop incredible strength.

Ed Lippie is a former collegiate football player, a strength coach, and a personal trainer, and he was a model for many of the pictures in the first edition of *Functional Training for Sports*. More relative to this sidebar, Ed used the techniques described in this chapter to perform three chin-ups with 135 pounds (60 kg), the best I have seen in our facility.

Ben Bruno is another former MBSC employee who has become a bit of a YouTube phenomenon with his tremendous displays of strength. Ben progressed to 305 pounds (140 kg) for five reps in the rear-foot-elevated split squat, again using a simple periodization approach. Whether you are an Olympic athlete, a coach, or a trainer, the basics of progressive resistance and periodization produce dramatic results.

Exercise Classifications

Our upper body, lower body, and core exercises are classified according to one of three terms:

- Baseline
- Progression
- Regression

Baseline exercises are the general starting point for the average athlete. We identify subsequent exercises as either progressions or regressions. Athletes perform the baseline exercise for three weeks and then move to a progression of the exercise. However, athletes who experience difficulty with the baseline exercise, either because of injury or technical issues, are immediately regressed. This system of progressions and regressions is the key tool for proper exercise performance.

Progressions are steps forward from the baseline exercises and are numbered consecutively from easy to difficult. Progression can be as simple as adding load via progressive resistance, but progressions in difficulty can also be achieved by altering how body weight is used. A progression 3 exercise will be fairly difficult.

Regressions are numbered also, but in reverse order on the scale, from easy to easier to easiest. Therefore, a regression 3 exercise will be very simple.

The key is understanding that every exercise must be mastered before progressing, and mastery may entail the use of regressions from the baseline.

I tell our coaches that you need to like the way the exercise looks before adding load or progressing and that our system of regressions is based on the "eye test." Do you as a coach like the way it looks?

I love this quote from legendary track and field coach Boo Schexnayder: "The job is not to write workouts but to watch workouts."

It's easy to put stuff down on paper, and it should be just as easy to watch someone do the things you wrote and then decide whether to stick with the baseline or prescribe a regression. Your eyes will tell you.

Training Tools

Many coaches and athletes think that functional training consists of cute exercises done with stability balls and balance devices. This could not be further from the truth. True functional training revolves around body-weight training and progressive resistance exercise. Athletes should master body-weight exercises and then add progressively heavier external loads to these exercises. Watch a novice attempt to split-squat with just his body weight; the lack of balance is evident. What we call *balance* is really stabilizer strength. In most cases, additional external resistance is not initially needed as the athlete learns the patterns. What is needed is to master the pattern and *then* add resistance.

Think of functional training as being the opposite of dysfunctional training, or as physical therapist and Functional Movement Screen cofounder Gray Cook is fond of saying, adding strength to dysfunction. Essential to the concept of functional training is learning to move before you load. Evidence of dysfunctional training is seen in every gym in the United States as people attempt to simply move a load from point A to point B with technique that varies from questionable to unsafe.

Following is a brief overview of some key pieces of functional training equipment and some simple guidelines for how and when to use them.

Medicine Balls   One of the best tools available for power development, the medicine ball has enjoyed a huge resurgence in the past decade. Although medicine balls (see figure 4.1) have been around for centuries, they have become tools of the future. The medicine ball can be used for upper body power work through exercises such as chest passes, overhead throws, and slams, and it can be thrown for distance for total-body power work. The medicine ball, when combined with a masonry wall, is hands down the best tool for power training of the core and hip musculature. An entire section on training with the medicine ball is included in chapter 9.

Common sense must be used to prevent injury with the medicine ball. Athletes at our training facility do not perform partner drills that require catching the ball, nor do they perform any single-arm overhead medicine ball movements. Catching a medicine ball can result in hand injury, while

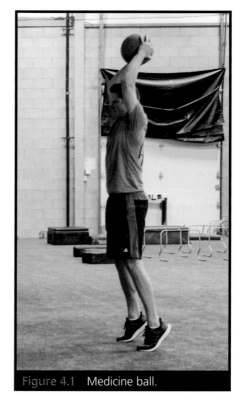

Figure 4.1   Medicine ball.

single-arm overhead activities may be too stressful on the shoulder joint. Balls come in bouncing and nonbouncing varieties and various weights and sizes. The most useful balls tend to be between 2 and 8 pounds (1 to 3.5 kg).

Weight Vests and Belts   There may not be a better tool for functional training than a weighted vest or belt. Weighted vests and belts are available in numerous styles and have come a long way from the old canvas fishing-style varieties. Some coaches may think that using a weighted vest or belt is redundant if athletes are already training with bars or dumbbells. However, a weighted vest adds an external load with minimal disruption of the movement of the body. Athletes do not need to change the position of the upper body to hold an external load; they simply need to put on a weighted vest or belt.

Vests and belts are excellent ways to add additional resistance to what were formerly viewed as body-weight exercises. Exercises such as push-ups, single-leg squats, and inverted rows can now be safely progressed well beyond body-weight resistance. In addition, for sports such as ice hockey and football, weighted vests and belts allow athletes to simulate the weight of equipment during conditioning workouts.

Foam Rollers   Foam rollers (see figure 4.2) have gone from a complete unknown to a must-have in the last decade. Rollers come in various colors, lengths, and densities but are all used for self-massage. The terms *self-myofascial release*, *self-massage*, and *soft tissue work* all apply to the act of foam rolling. Chapter 5 covers the use of the roller in great detail.

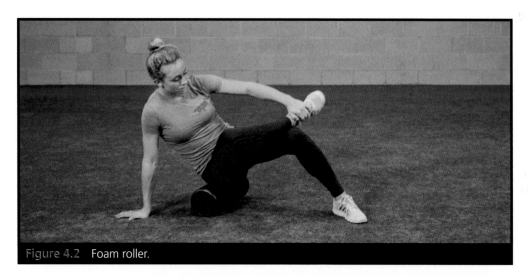

Figure 4.2   Foam roller.

Stability Balls   The stability ball (see figure 4.3) has unfortunately become synonymous with functional training, with books, videos, and classes all developed around this one piece of equipment. The overuse of the stability ball alone has caused many strength and conditioning coaches to view the entire area of functional training negatively. Coaches and athletes need to remember that it is simply one tool and may be inappropriate for many beginning trainees. The stability ball is excellent for a few specific exercises (e.g., stability ball rollouts, stability ball leg curls), but it is far from the training panacea it was initially viewed as, and it is certainly not a tool for squatting or for lifting loads heavier than body weight. Videos showing athletes standing on a ball are negligent. Athletes should never stand on a stability ball. The risks far outweigh any potential benefits. If you desire an unstable surface for additional balance training for the lower extremity, use another tool.

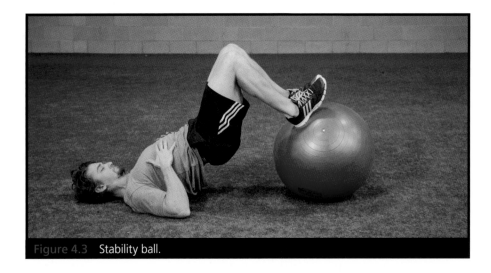

Figure 4.3   Stability ball.

Coaches and athletes should also be cautious about sitting on a stability ball during barbell or dumbbell exercises or using the stability ball as a substitute for a bench for pressing movements. Stability balls should never be used for support when using dumbbells or a bar. Caution should even be used with so called burst-resistant balls. There have been reports of burst-resistant balls tearing in the same manner as conventional balls and causing serious injury. Our current policy is body weight only and no standing on stability balls for safety reasons.

Slide Board   The slide board was initially developed as a training device for speedskaters, but its use is now widespread in other sports. The slide board allows the athlete to perform energy system work while standing and, by its nature, forces athletes to assume the bent-knee posture that has been dubbed the sport-specific position (see figure 4.4). It is the only piece of conditioning equipment that can provide energy system and muscular system work in this position. Athletes can develop conditioning while also developing appropriate muscle patterns, something that is usually not possible on a conventional piece of cardiorespiratory equipment.

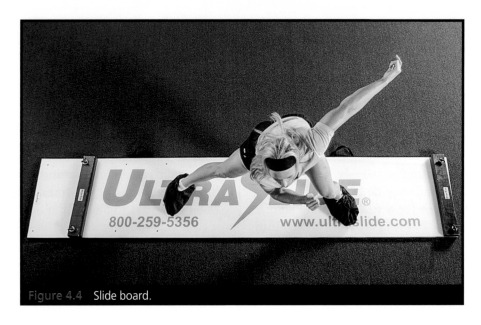

Figure 4.4   Slide board.

The slide board allows the athlete to work all the extensor muscles of the lower body as well as the hip abductors and adductors. From a functional conditioning standpoint, the benefits of the slide board may be equal to or better than running.

At our training facility, we require all our athletes to use the slide board, as it can enhance lateral movement and balance while also conditioning the difficult-to-train hip abductor and adductor muscle groups. No other piece of energy system conditioning equipment can provide all these benefits. In addition, the slide board can easily accommodate users of various heights and weights.

Mini Slide Board   The mini slide board has no bumpers but can be used for lower body exercises such as slide-board lunges and slide-board leg curls and for a wide range of core progressions. It is not a slide board in the conventional sense because you cannot perform energy system work on it, but it is still a great tool to have in the toolbox.

Valslides   Invented by L.A. trainer to the stars Valerie Waters, the Valslide allows for mini slide-board-type exercise on any carpeted or turf surface. Like the mini slide board, the Valslide can be used for lower body and core work.

Agility Ladder   The agility ladder may be one of the best pieces of functional training equipment available. It allows a dynamic warm-up that can emphasize any number of components, and it can be used to develop balance, foot speed, coordination, and eccentric strength (see figure 4.5). Until the advent of the agility ladder, there was no good way to work on foot speed. The agility ladder provides benefits to both the muscular system and the neuromuscular system while increasing muscle temperature.

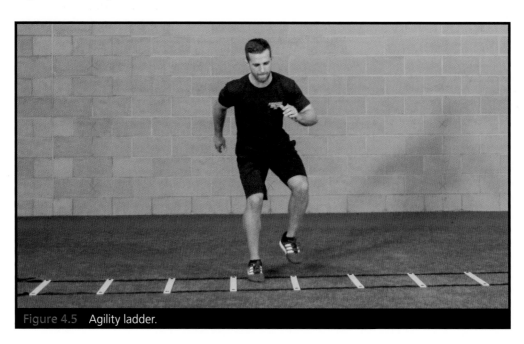

Figure 4.5   Agility ladder.

BOSU Ball   The BOSU ball makes the list for only one reason: It is an excellent tool for adding upper body instability to the push-up and offers an excellent progression from feet-elevated push-ups. We keep BOSU balls in the facility just for push-ups.

Suspension Trainers   Suspension trainers have become very popular over the last decade. The TRX is the most popular commercial model, but there are many varieties. I have become a fan of rings for suspension training more than the TRX, and the reality is that like the BOSU ball, we use our TRX or rings for only one exercise, inverted rows. Suspension trainers make inverted rows better for two major reasons. First, the TRX and rings are adjustable so you can make a challenging row for athletes or clients at any level. Second, a suspension trainer allows the shoulders to begin internally rotated (thumbs down) and end externally rotated (thumbs up). This creates a very shoulder-friendly exercise.

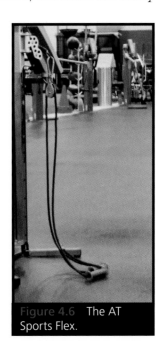

Figure 4.6   The AT Sports Flex.

AT Sports Flex   It's rare that a piece of equipment this simple could so drastically affect how we do certain exercises. The AT Sports Flex (see figure 4.6) is a multifunction cable attachment that is great for presses, rows, and scapulothoracic work. Its design is so unique that I would consider it an essential tool. Developed by Chicago White Sox strength and conditioning coach Allen Thomas (hence the *AT*), this piece is a must-have.

THE FUNCTIONAL CONTINUUM

Given the importance of determining the functional properties of an exercise or drill when designing a program, I thought it would be useful to have a taxonomy to refer to in this regard. The functional continuum (see figure 4.7) evaluates exercises on a scale that moves from least functional to most functional.

This chart is divided into lower body exercises (both knee dominant and hip dominant), upper body exercises (both pushing and pulling), and core exercises. The figure depicts the progression from the relatively nonfunctional machine-based exercises to highly functional exercises done on a single leg. This schematic reinforces the notion that program design should be thought of not in either/or terms but rather as an integrated approach to developing strength and making that strength more relevant to sport and movement.

The continuum shown in the figure, from least functional to most functional, is of knee-dominant lower-body exercises. And it follows this sequence:

1. The least functional exercise I could envision is a lying leg press. In the leg press, the athlete is lying on his back, and stability is provided by the machine.

2. Next comes the standing machine squat. The athlete has progressed up the functional continuum to a standing position, which is an improvement, but the machine is still providing the stability and the stance remains bilateral.

3. Then it is on to the barbell squat. At this point the athlete is standing and self-stabilizing, but the exercise is still not at the highest level of function.

4. The next step in the progression is to work on one leg: a single-leg squat. At this point the exercise is extremely functional. The muscles of the lower body and trunk are now engaged as they would be in running or jumping.

Least functional ➡ Most functional				
Lower body exercises				
Knee-dominant				
Type of exercise	Leg press	Machine squat	Barbell squat	Rear-foot-elevated split squat	One-leg squat
Rationale	Lying, no stabilization by athlete	Standing, no stabilization by athlete	Two legs	One leg, additional balance assistance	One leg with no additional balance assistance
Hip-dominant				
Type of exercise	Leg curl	Back extension	Two-leg SLDL or RDL*	One-leg SLDL* with 2 DB	One-leg SLDL* with 1 DB
Rationale	Prone, non-functional action	Prone, functional action	Standing on two legs	Standing on one leg	Standing on one leg with glute/lumbar connection
Upper body exercises				
Horizontal press				
Type of exercise	Machine bench press	Bench press	Dumbbell bench press	Push-up	Stability-ball push-up
Rationale	Supine, no stabilization by athlete	Supine, moderate stabilization	Supine, single-arm stabilization	Prone with closed chain	Prone with additional challenge to balance
Horizontal pull				
Type of exercise	Machine row	Dumbbell row	Inverted row	One-arm, one-leg row	One-arm, two-leg rotational row
Torso exercises				
Type of exercise	Crunch	In-line half-kneeling lift	Lunge position lift	Standing lift	Medicine ball side throw
Rationale	Lying, no rotation	Half-kneeling lift with limited core movement	Lunge position with limited core movement	Standing with weight stack and IR/ER	Standing with explosive movement

* SLDL = Straight-leg deadlift; RDL = Romanian deadlift (modified straight-leg deadlift)

Figure 4.7 The functional continuum.

FUNCTIONAL TRAINING AND FEMALE ATHLETES

Trainers and coaches are always curious how training should differ between male and female athletes. Often coaches pose questions that begin or end with "but I coach women." Female athletes are not physically different from their male counterparts, at least not as it relates to training. All muscles and bones are the same. Any differences really have no bearing on how a training program would be designed or applied. At no point should coaches lower their expectations for female athletes. Most of what I was initially told about training female athletes proved to be untrue. Whether this is unintentional is not clear, but most preconceptions about training female athletes are not accurate.

The old theory that female athletes need to stay away from body-weight upper body exercises is particularly untrue. What holds female athletes back is often the low expectations and preconceptions of those training them. Women and girls may not be able to begin with a body-weight exercise such as the chin-up, but they are able to progress to it quickly. After training elite female athletes in basketball, soccer, field hockey, ice hockey, and figure skating, we have found that they are easily able to perform push-ups and chin-ups when they are progressed properly. Although they may not possess the same upper body strength as elite male athletes, they can develop excellent upper body strength.

Female athletes are often no more flexible than male athletes in similar sports. Our elite women's ice hockey players suffer from the same tightness in the hips that our men do. Our elite female soccer players are not significantly more flexible than their male counterparts. Athletes develop tightness and inflexibility based on the repetitive patterns of their sports, not on sex.

Women are more coachable and not as extrinsically competitive as men. By extrinsically competitive, I mean that women are not nearly as worried about what another athlete is lifting. Women tend to focus more on what they can do and less on what others are doing. This makes them easier to coach.

But body image is a huge issue for female athletes, who are much more concerned about not building muscle than male athletes are. This is a unique societal influence that coaches must be aware of and work to overcome. Statistics about weight and body fat percentages are often fabricated, inflated, or deflated and provide unrealistic expectations for female athletes. The only body fat information given to athletes should come from the coach, sports medicine staff, or exercise science department. Comparing the body composition of athletes at other schools or in other programs done with different methods, at different times, by different people is comparing apples and oranges. Female athletes must be reminded of what height and weight is normal for their sport and their body type.

Some athletic programs have adopted a head-in-the-sand approach to issues of eating disorders, body image, and nutrition by prohibiting coaches from weighing or measuring their female athletes. This does a great disservice to these women. The solution is addressing the issues, not avoiding them. Education and the promotion of positive role models are essential for female athletes.

Female athletes need to be exposed to photos of athletes similar to themselves who have a body composition that is considered acceptable. All too often visual role models for women are fashion models or entertainers who do not have the attributes of the average female athlete.

OVERCOMING THE FEMALE BODY IMAGE ISSUE

Just after the 2012 Winter Olympics, U.S. women's national team hockey player Hilary Knight appeared in the famed *ESPN The Magazine's* body issue at a body weight of 172 pounds (79 kg). When the first edition of *Functional Training for Sports* was published, I'm not sure any female athlete would have admitted to being 172 pounds. I knew tour players in women's tennis who regularly lied about their weight in the media. Knight was quoted as saying: "There is this image of athletic women as small and petite—the yoga body type. Women in general, we tend

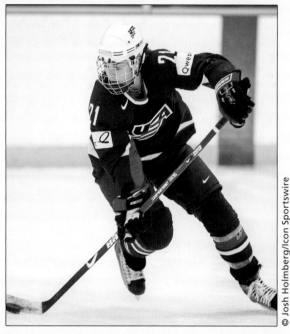

© Josh Holmberg/Icon Sportswire

to shrink ourselves and not have as much confidence as we should in presenting ourselves and our body types. It's OK to be fit and healthy and comfortable within your body, whatever frame you have. Since gaining 15 pounds to be at the top of my sport [for the Olympics], I've tried to shatter the body image that muscular isn't feminine."

The truth is that I convinced Hilary to get bigger, stronger, and faster to become the best in the world. Little did I know that our programing would also be creating one of the most beautiful examples of what a female athlete can and should look like. For too long female athletes were ashamed to list their actual weight for fear they would be perceived as fat. An athlete like Hilary in the body issues tells thousands of young girls that it's OK to be a female athlete.

When you design a program, it is important to note that the most functional exercise is often not the most appropriate exercise. Instead, follow the progressions outlined in this book, master the basics, and strive to develop great functional strength by the end of the program. These are the key points:

- Learn the basics.
- Use body weight first.
- Progress from simple to complex.

I have a simple rule: Everything has to look good. Exercises should look smooth and athletic. If athletes are struggling to master an exercise, they should go back a level and work toward mastery. Technique comes before all else, and always before the amount of weight lifted.

Equipment Needs for Training Female Athletes

The major differences for training women and girls actually center around equipment needs and progression. Most personal trainers and strength coaches do not consider the unique equipment needs of female athletes.

All the following recommendations also apply to training young athletes of either sex.

■ *15-, 25-, and 35-pound (7, 11, and 16 kg) Olympic bars.* Many young and female athletes have little or no strength training background and may need lighter bars to begin with. Buy lighter Olympic bars that take Olympic plates. Many companies now stock these new lighter, shorter bars. Also, don't use conventional bars and one-inch-hole plates. Purchase full-size plastic plates that are the size of a regulation 45-pound (20 kg) plate. Younger and weaker athletes should look like everyone else in the weight room. Seeing themselves in the mirror with large-diameter plates provides a huge psychological boost.

■ *Dumbbells in 2.5-pound increments.* Dumbbells in 2.5-pound (1 kg) increments are ideal for younger athletes and female athletes. Five-pound (2.5 kg) increments do not allow younger or less-trained athletes to progress at reasonable rates. Consider that when less-experienced athletes advance from two 15-pound (7 kg) dumbbells to two 20-pound (10 kg) dumbbells, they are progressing from 30 pounds (15 kg) to 40 pounds (20 kg), an increase of 33 percent. Would you ask a stronger athlete to go from 60-pound (30 kg) dumbbells to 90-pound (40 kg) dumbbells in one week? Having dumbbells from 5 through at least 50 in 2.5-pound increments is essential.

■ *1.25-pound PlateMates.* If you have only 5-pound-increment dumbbells, PlateMates are the solution. PlateMates are simply 1.25-pound (.6 kg) magnets that allow you to increase a dumbbell's weight by 2.5 pounds (one PlateMate on each side). Make sure to purchase the proper PlateMates for your style of dumbbell: hexagonal or round. Round PlateMates do not work well on hexagonal dumbbells and could pose a safety hazard.

■ *1.25-pound Olympic plates.* These are not common but can be purchased. The same logic described earlier applies. Moving from 45 pounds to 50 pounds is only a 5-pound jump, but it is also a 10 percent jump. Many female athletes will not be able to make this type of progression. The male example again illustrates this point. Ask a male athlete to jump from 300 to 330 on the bench press in one week. This is only a 10 percent jump, but it would be impossible for any athlete.

■ *Dip belts.* As your athletes gain strength, they can start to perform weighted chin-ups and possibly weighted dips. Conventional dip belts can fall off small female athletes. Belts need to be custom made to fit a female athlete's waist.

■ *Weight belts.* Again most weight rooms are outfitted with weight belts. If you are a proponent of weight belts, purchase some size 24 to 28 belts for the females. This is one clear area of difference. Females generally have smaller waists than males.

Once your facility is properly equipped, functional training for female athletes does not present any problems. With proper equipment, female athletes can use all the functional training concepts discussed in this book, and their training programs will have most of the characteristics of programs for male athletes. One possible exception is the use of body weight as the initial resistance for upper body work. Exercises such as push-ups and pull-ups may need to be modified for beginning female athletes. Although women and girls can develop excellent upper body strength, they may not have it to begin with. However, body-weight exercises can easily be modified for the female population.

REFERENCES

Poliquin, C. 1988. Variety in strength training. *Science Periodical on Research and Technology in Sport.* 8 (8): 1-7.

Foam Rolling, Stretching, and Dynamic Warm-Up

With regard to the prescription of pre- and posttraining activities and apparatuses, you can be assured of one thing: It will continue to change and improve as a more functional vantage point permeates sports training. The old days of performing a series of the same static stretches for every sport, just because, doesn't cut it anymore.

FOAM ROLLING

A degree of skepticism is warranted when it comes to new training equipment and gadgets. For every one useful innovation, three or four others are junk not deserving even a minute on one of those late-night infomercials. And yet, we also need to be receptive to inventions and creative solutions, despite how strange they may seem initially.

When the first edition of *Functional Training for Sports* was published in 2004 we had not even begun to use a foam roller in our preworkout sequence. In fact, 10 years ago strength and conditioning coaches, athletic trainers, and physical therapists would have looked quizzically at a round 36-inch (90 cm) piece of foam and asked a simple question: *What am I supposed to do with that?*

Today nearly every strength and conditioning facility contains an array of foam rollers, foam balls, lacrosse balls, and plastic peanuts in different lengths and consistencies, all designed for self-massage. We have hard rollers, soft rollers, rollers with protrusions. The array of soft tissue tools is amazing and increases every year. What turned a simple piece of foam into a must-have preparation tool?

What happened was that strength and conditioning coaches and personal trainers began to realize that massage might be the fastest way to get healthy and stay healthy. This major change in the attitude toward injury prevention and treatment has been illustrated by a huge increase in the awareness that hands-on techniques such as conventional massage, Muscle Activation Techniques (MAT), and Active Release Techniques (ART) can work wonders for injured athletes.

We have moved away from the injury care modes of isokinetics and electronics that were popular in the 1980s to a more European-inspired process that focuses on hands-on soft tissue care. The success of physical therapists with soft tissue mobilization (the physical therapy term for massage) and MAT, and a number of chiropractors with ART, has clearly put the focus back on the quality of the muscle. The message from the elite levels of sport is clear: If you want to get healthy or stay healthy, get a good manual therapist in your corner.

What does all this have to do with foam rollers, you might ask? Well, foam rollers are the poor man's answer to a good massage therapist, offering soft tissue work for the masses. As strength and conditioning coaches and personal trainers watched elite-level athletes tout their successes and improvements from various soft tissue techniques, the obvious question arose: How can we mass-produce massage or soft tissue work for large groups of athletes at a reasonable cost? Enter the foam roller.

Physical therapist Mike Clark is credited by many, this author included, with exposing the athletic and physical therapy communities to the foam roller and to what he termed "self-myofascial release." Self-myofascial release is simply another technical term for self-massage.

One of Clark's early manuals, published as a precursor to his book *Integrated Training for the New Millennium*, included a few photos of these so-called self-myofascial release techniques using a foam roller. The techniques illustrated were simple and fairly self-explanatory. Get a foam roller and use body weight to apply pressure to sore spots. It was a form of a self-acupressure.

A MINUTE ABOUT MASSAGE

I believe that massage fell out of favor during the physical therapy boom of the 1980s not because it was ineffective, but because it was not cost effective. With the increased use of modalities such as ultrasound and electrical stimulation, athletic trainers and physical therapists could treat more athletes, more rapidly. In Europe and in certain elite-level sports, such as track and field and swimming, massage remained the preference over modality-based solutions. Slowly, the performance world has come to appreciate that manipulation of the soft tissue helps athletes either stay healthier or get healthy faster.

The use of foam rollers has progressed from an acupressure-type approach to a self-massage approach. The roller is now used to apply longer, more sweeping strokes to the long muscle groups such as the calves, adductors, and quadriceps and smaller, more directed force to areas such as the tensor fasciae latae (TFL), hip rotators, and gluteus medius. Rollers come in various sizes, thicknesses, and densities and have spawned a whole generation of other soft tissue tools. Athletes now use rollers as well as balls, sticks, and even in some cases PVC pipe.

Using the foam roller before stretching makes the tissue more pliable and extensible. The key is to search for tender areas, or trigger points, and to roll these areas to decrease tissue density and overactivity. Tissue that has been rolled can elongate properly. Why rolling works remains a controversial topic, but no one seems to doubt that it does work. Most athletes or clients, even those initially skeptical, are quickly converted to foam roller fans.

It is important to note that foam rolling is very counterintuitive. We have consistently told our clients "if it hurts, don't do it." Foam rolling is the opposite. We are now encouraging our clients to find the sore spots and focus on them. Foam rolling probably falls into the "hurts so good" category.

Those photos spurred a trend that is now probably a multimillion-dollar business in the manufacture and sale of these simple tools. Suddenly the warm-up was not literally about temperature (think about the term *warm-up*) but about muscle tissue quality. Muscle tissue, and the joints that muscles control, has to be properly prepared for any activity. Muscle tissue that is filled with knots, adhesions, or trigger points (three different words that describe the same thing) may not function optimally even when warmed.

Using a Foam Roller

A foam roller is simply a cylindrical piece of some type of extruded hard-celled foam. Think pool noodles but a little more dense and larger in diameter.

Mike Clark's initial recommendation was not even a self-massage technique but more like the acupressure concept described previously. Athletes or patients were simply instructed to use the roller to apply pressure to sensitive areas in the muscles. Depending on the orientation of the therapist, these points can alternatively be described as trigger points, knots, or simply areas of increased muscle density. Regardless of the name, those in the fields of athletics and rehab were familiar with the concepts of sore muscles and the need for massage.

The Rationale for Foam Rolling

Trying to explain the "why" of foam rolling centers around two concepts:

1. creep and
2. a pair of terms that rolfer Thomas Myers coined, *locked long* and *locked short*.

Creep is a property common to extensible soft tissues. They become stiffer as they are extended due to the reorientation of collagen fibers (Currier and Nelson 1992). Mechanical creep is defined as elongation of tissue beyond its intrinsic extensibility, resulting from a constant load over time (Wilhelmi et al. 1998).

The analogy I often use to describe creep involves slowly pushing a fist into a plastic bag. If the pressure is slow and consistent the bag does not tear immediately but instead stretches from the constant load over time. Think about sitting. One study by noted back pain researcher Stuart McGill concluded that "sitting with the back slouched for as little as 20 minutes can result in increased laxity of the posterior spinal ligaments" (McGill and Brown 1992). The result of creep is a change in the quality of the muscle tissue, or the fascia. In either case the tissue becomes what Thomas Myers refers to as "locked long."

"Stretched, a muscle will attempt to recoil back to its resting length before giving up and adding more cells and sarcomeres to bridge the gap. Stretch fascia quickly and it will tear (the most frequent form of connective tissue injury). If the stretch is applied slowly enough, it will deform plastically: it will change its length and retain that change" (Myers 2009, 36).

The important point about creep is that these constant low-load forces caused by sitting make muscle tissue (or the superficial fascia) longer and more dense. We see an increase in collagen and effectively tissue that is locked long. Think of foam rolling as a way to combat creep.

We most often see creep in the back side of the body, in the upper and lower back, glutes, and hamstrings. These are also the areas that seem to benefit most from the foam roller. In simple terms, we need to roll the back side of the body (but not stretch because it is already lengthened) and then roll and stretch the front side.

So, which is a better way to combat creep, massage therapy or foam rolling? To me the answer is obvious. Hands work better than foam. Hands are directly connected to the brain and can feel. A foam roller cannot feel. If cost were not an issue I would have a team of massage therapists on call for my athletes at all times.

However, this is simply not realistic. Most athletes struggle to afford the services of a qualified coach or the cost of a gym membership. In the current state of health care, prevention is generally not a covered cost for healthy athletes. With no ability to get reimbursed, the cost of massage therapy alone could approach or surpass the cost of training. The foam roller can provide unlimited self-massage for under 20 dollars. You do the math.

Foam Rolling Techniques and Tips

Rolling can provide great benefits both before and after a workout; however, rolling at the start of a workout is essential. Foam rolling before a workout decreases muscle density and sets the stage for a better warm-up. Rolling after a workout may aid in recovery from strenuous exercise. The nice thing about the foam roller is that it can be used on a daily basis. In fact, Clair and Amber Davies recommend trigger point work up to 12 times a day in situations of acute pain (2004).

How long an athlete or client rolls is also individual. In our setting we allow 5 to 10 minutes for soft tissue work at the beginning of the session before the warm-up.

Let's now look at the primary areas of the body where athletes most benefit from foam rolling and the techniques used to get the best results. Although there are no hard and fast rules, a general rule of thumb is to do 10 slow rolls in each position. Often athletes or clients are encouraged to simply roll until the pain dissipates or disappears.

▶ FOAM ROLLING THE GLUTEUS MAXIMUS AND HIP ROTATORS

The hip rotators sit below the glutes. To roll the hips the athlete sits on the roller with a slight tilt toward the side to be rolled and moves from the iliac crest to the hip joint to address the glute max. To address the hip rotators more specifically, the leg is crossed to place the hip rotator group on stretch (see figure 5.1).

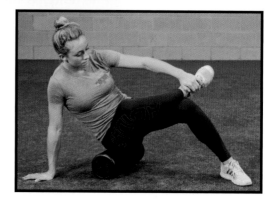

Figure 5.1   Gluteus maximus and hip rotators.

FOAM ROLLING THE LOW BACK

After rolling the hips, the athlete rolls the lower back area (see figure 5.2), tilting slightly right or left to get into the spinal erectors and quadratus lumborum, a large triangular muscle layered under the spinal erectors. If you have any concerns about spinal injury, skip the low back. We have never had any issues with rolling the lumbar spine, but use common sense and proceed with caution.

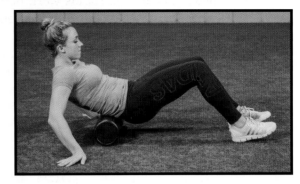

Figure 5.2 Low back.

FOAM ROLLING THE UPPER BACK

The athlete moves up the body, continuing to roll the spinal erectors, the large layers of muscle on either side of the spine. When the athlete reaches the area between the shoulder blades, instruct him to try to touch the elbows together in front to get into the area known as the thoracic spine (see figure 5.3). Putting the elbows together places the shoulder blades as far apart as possible, allowing the roller to impact the lower trapezius and rhomboids.

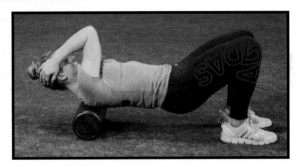

Figure 5.3 Upper back.

FOAM ROLLING THE TENSOR FASCIAE LATAE AND GLUTEUS MEDIUS

The TFL and gluteus medius, although small muscles, can be significant factors in anterior knee pain. To address the TFL the athlete begins with the body prone and the edge of the roller placed over the TFL, just below the iliac crest (see figure 5.4a). After working the TFL, the athlete turns 90 degrees to a side position and works from the hip joint to the iliac crest to address the gluteus medius (see figure 5.4b).

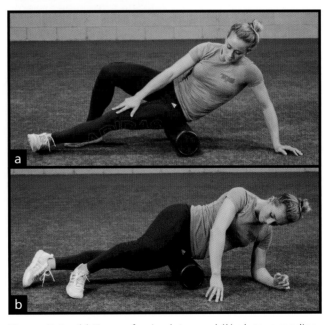

Figure 5.4 (a) Tensor fasciae latae and (b) gluteus medius.

▶ FOAM ROLLING THE ADDUCTORS

The adductors are probably the most neglected area of the lower body. A great deal of time and energy is focused on the quadriceps and hamstring groups and very little attention paid to the adductors. There are two methods to roll the adductors. The first is a floor-based technique that works well for beginners (see figure 5.5). In the floor technique the user abducts the leg over the roller and places the roller at about a 60-degree angle to the leg. The rolling action should cover three portions beginning just above the knee in the area of the vastus medialis and pes anserine. The athlete does 10 short rolls, covering about one-third the length of the femur. Next, she moves the roller to the midpoint of the adductor group and again rolls 10 times in the middle third of the muscle. Last, she moves the roller high into the groin, almost to the pubic symphysis.

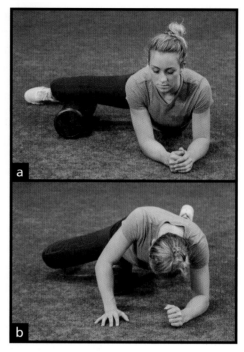

Figure 5.5 Adductors.

The secondary technique for the adductors should be used after the athlete has acclimated to the previous technique. The secondary technique requires a training room table or the top of a plyometric box. Sitting with the leg dropped over the roller allows the athlete to shift significantly more weight onto the roller and work deeper into the large adductor triangle.

▶ FOAM ROLLING THE POSTERIOR SHOULDER

Another area in need of work is the posterior shoulder. To roll the posterior shoulder, the athlete lies on the side with the arm draped over the roller (see figure 5.6). The rolling action is slightly side to side while rolling to a facedown position and then back to faceup. This will impact the lat and rotator cuff muscles.

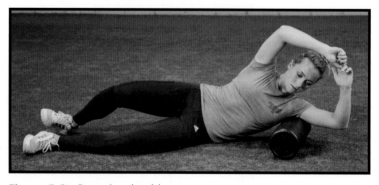

Figure 5.6 Posterior shoulder.

FOAM ROLLING THE PECS

The last area to hit with the roller is the pectorals, or chest muscles. To roll the pecs, the athlete lies facedown with the roller nearly parallel to the body and the arm draped over the roller (see figure 5.7). Males can roll side to side in a short stroke. Females will do better simply raising the arm overhead and back in a reaching motion.

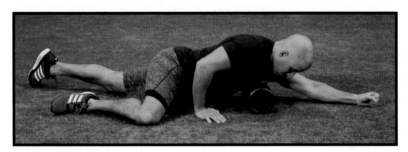

Figure 5.7   Pecs.

Foam rolling can be hard work, particularly for weaker or overweight athletes, as the arms are heavily involved in moving the body. In addition, foam rolling can border on painful. Good massage work, and correspondingly good self-massage work, may be uncomfortable, much like stretching. It is important that athletes or clients learn to distinguish between a moderate level of discomfort related to a trigger point and a potentially injurious situation. Foam rolling should be used with discretion in those athletes or clients with less muscle density. It should never cause bruising. Remember, the athlete or client should feel better, not worse after a brief session with a foam roller.

Rollers are available in a number of densities, from relatively soft foam, slightly harder than a pool noodle, to newer high-density rollers with a much more solid feel. The feel of the roller and the intensity of the self-massage work must be properly geared to the age and fitness level of the client.

The use of foam rollers has exploded over the past 10 years and will continue to increase. Athletic trainers in high schools and colleges can teach their athletes to perform hands-on treatment that might not otherwise have been possible, while strength and conditioning coaches can provide a form of massage therapy to all their athletes. Foam rollers are a small investment to make to see a potentially significant decrease in the number of noncontact soft tissue injuries.

STATIC STRETCHING

In the field of strength and conditioning the pendulum never stops swinging. In the first edition *of Functional Training for Sports* we specifically said not to stretch before exercise. Ten years later, all our athletes and clients now stretch before every workout.

Performance enhancement expert Alwyn Cosgrove is fond of saying we overreact in the short term and underreact in the long term to new ideas. In other words, we quickly jump on a trend and just as quickly abandon it.

A classic example is the use of or disdain for static stretching. Static stretching has gone from the best way to warm up to something no one should ever do again. We have seen the pendulum swing from whole teams on the ground stretching before practice to situations where no one is allowed to stretch before practice. The reaction to static stretching perfectly illustrates Cosgrove's short-term overreaction and long-term underreaction.

Research in the 1980s demonstrated that static stretching before exercise could decrease muscular power output. This led to a huge overreaction, the elimination of static stretching, and the birth of the dynamic warm-up. This was both a plus and a minus.

Dynamic flexibility work has been a huge plus in the performance world as a warm-up technique. Static stretching is a poor way to warm up for exercise, but it is still necessary for long-term injury prevention. Dynamic flexibility work, or an active warm-up, is superior before exercise. However, the effect of the research showing decreases in power led to total disdain for static stretching at any time, for any purpose. The truth lies somewhere in the middle.

One side of the truth is that an active warm-up before high-intensity exercise is the best way to prevent acute injury. In other words, if you want to decrease hamstring and groin pulls, you need to perform dynamic flexibility exercises before practices, games, or lifting sessions.

However, there is also truth on the other side of the coin. A lack of flexibility seems to be a causative factor in many of the gradual-onset injuries that plague today's athletes. Overuse problems such as patellofemoral syndrome, low back pain, and shoulder pain seem to relate strongly to long-term tissue changes that don't necessarily respond to dynamic stretching.

The fact is that athletes' warm-ups need to be a combination of both active warm-up exercises and static stretching, all preceded by foam rolling. For many coaches, the solution was seen as active warm-up before exercise and static stretching after. Although this seems realistic, the thought process is somewhat flawed. Postworkout stretching does not seem to produce gains in flexibility.

The key may lie in performing static stretching near the beginning of the workout, *followed by* dynamic warm-up. Static stretching would be done to increase flexibility while the muscle is most prone to increase in length. Dynamic warm-up should follow to prepare the muscles for exercise. Coaches need to think about length changes for long-term injury prevention and dynamic warm-up for short-term injury prevention. Both are critical.

Therefore, our prescription is as follows:

1. *Foam rolling.* Use the foam roller techniques previously presented for 5 to 10 minutes to decrease the density of the muscle. Muscles respond to injury, overuse, or overstress (creep) by increasing in density. This increased density is often referred to as a knot or trigger point. Massage, Active Release Techniques (ART), Muscle Activation Techniques (MAT), and soft tissue mobilization are all terms for techniques designed to change muscle density. I like to think of foam rolling as ironing for the muscles, a necessary precursor to stretching.

2. *Static stretching.* Yes, static stretching. Yes, before the workout. Once the tissue density has been dealt with, you can work on changing the length. Many top soft tissue experts are now recommending that muscles be stretched "cold," without the benefit of a warm-up. Simply roll and stretch. The theory is that warm muscle simply elongates and returns to its normal length. Cold muscle may in fact undergo some plastic deformation and increase in length. I like static stretches that make it easy for athletes to stretch. One reason athletes don't like to stretch is that it's hard. Stretches that allow an athlete to use body weight and positioning to their advantage are a big plus for athletes. Partner stretches can also be good.

3. *Dynamic warm-up.* This is done after rolling and stretching. Any potential power decreases should be negated by the dynamic warm-up that follows a static stretch. The process for my athletes every day is the same. Foam rolling to decrease knots and trigger points. Static stretching to work on increasing flexibility. Follow that up with a dynamic warm-up.

Static Stretching Rules

- Positioning is everything. Be specific about how you stretch. Most people don't stretch; they just try to look as if they are stretching.
- Good stretching is uncomfortable but not painful. Know the difference. A little discomfort means you are well positioned.
- Use different techniques. Activate the antagonist; do long, static stretches; use active stretches.
- Use body weight to assist. Be both comfortable and uncomfortable at the same time.
- Stretch all areas. Don't focus on one. Include one stretch for each of the following areas:
  - Adductors
  - Hip flexors
  - Lateral hamstrings
  - Hip rotators

Carolina Hurricanes trainer and strength coach Peter Friesen has a theory. He thinks it is more dangerous to be overly flexible in one muscle group than to be tight in all of them. Athletes shouldn't just do the stretches they like or are good at. In fact, it might be a good idea to eliminate or abbreviate the ones they are good at and have them work harder on the ones they don't like.

Static Stretching Techniques and Tips

The bottom line is stretching is highly underrated. Athletes who want to be healthy long term need to add some old-fashioned stretching to their workouts. Another tip is to tie breathing into stretching.

For years I poked fun at yoga instructors and all the emphasis on breathing. Recent research has proven them right and me wrong. Breathing matters, and it matters a lot.

Tight athletes tend to hold their breath while stretching and probably create more tension. Think about holding a stretch for three breaths instead of for time. Instruct the athlete to inhale through the nose (yes, this matters because the nose is a natural filter that warms air) and exhale through the mouth. Strive for 1:2 ratio of inhale to exhale—a three-count inhale through the nose and a six-count exhale through the mouth. When exhaling we want the athletes to exhale through pursed lips (yes, this matters also).

STANDING HAMSTRING STRETCH

This stretch is best done on a training room table, large plyo box, or another area slightly below waist height (see figure 5.8).

Position

Keep both feet pointed straight forward. This is actually a neutral hip position. Think of the feet as images of the hips. If the feet turn in, the hip internally rotates.

Action

The hamstrings don't attach to the spine, they attach to the pelvis. So to stretch the hamstrings, move the pelvis, don't flex the spine. This is so difficult that we often have to manually teach athletes how to do this.

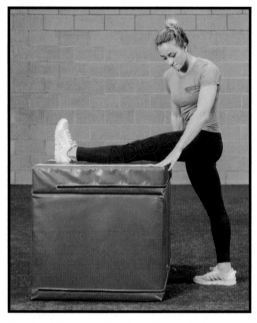

Figure 5.8   Standing hamstring stretch.

WALL HAMSTRING STRETCH

I love this stretch because it takes no effort. The key is to position correctly (see figure 5.9).

Position

Find the perfect distance from the wall—the butt is on the floor and there is a slight lumbar arch. Ideally place a small lumbar roll under the low back to maintain a small lordosis. Remember, the hamstrings insert to the pelvis, not the spine.

Action

Get the toes and ankles to touch. As stated previously, most tightness is lateral, or outside. External hip rotation will be comfortable; work for neutral or ideally internal rotation to properly stretch the lateral structures.

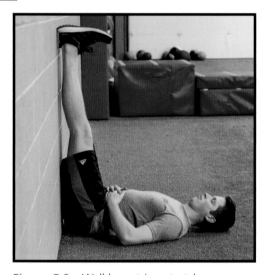

Figure 5.9   Wall hamstring stretch.

ROLLER HIP FLEXOR STRETCH

The anterior hip structures (iliacus and psoas) are the most difficult muscles to stretch. Most hip flexor stretches actually miss the hip flexors and apply excessive stress to the anterior hip capsule. To effectively stretch the hip flexors, the lumbar spine must be kept flat. Extending the spine actually shortens the psoas rather than lengthens it. The addition of a foam roller between the legs allows a better position to begin the stretch and encourages spinal flexion versus spinal extension.

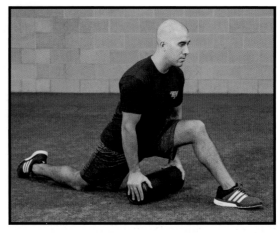

Figure 5.10   Roller hip flexor stretch.

Position

To perform this stretch, straddle the roller and attempt to do a split (see figure 5.10). This will be difficult, but the roller makes it possible for most athletes. From this position simply bend the front leg while attempting to straighten the back leg.

Action

Use the arms for support and to reduce pressure. Think about firing the back-side glute as this will have a direct impact on the psoas stretch.

BOX HIP FLEXOR STRETCH

This is the best hip flexor stretch we have found. The addition of a six-inch (15 cm) box under the front foot and a starting position that drives the hip into internal rotation are the keys. The box creates greater flexion of the hip and stabilizes the lumbar spine. Positioning the body at 45 degrees to the box and then internally rotating to get the foot on the box drives internal rotation of the down (stretched) leg.

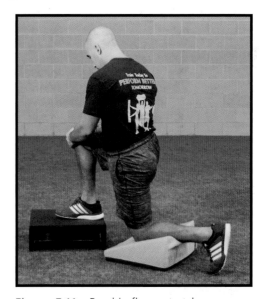

Position

Begin with the left knee down and the right foot on the floor, not the box. The body should be at 45 degrees to the box (see figure 5.11). From here place the right foot up on the box. Doing this will force internal rotation of the left hip as the pelvis rotates.

Figure 5.11   Box hip flexor stretch.

Action

Think slight posterior pelvic tilt to effect the psoas body on the lumbar spine. The right foot should be positioned slightly outside of the right hip. This is key because the iliacus and psoas attachments are on the inside of the femur, and the hip internal rotation will create a greater length change.

MOBILITY AND ACTIVATION

Mobility and activation exercises weren't addressed in the first edition of *Functional Training for Sports*. In fact, the words *flexibility* and *mobility* were probably considered interchangeable 10 years ago. The joint-by-joint approach to training helped change that. To fully understand the joint-by-joint approach you must understand that, as famed physical therapist Stanley Paris says, "pain never precedes dysfunction." You must also understand that the goal of functional training is to prevent or repair dysfunction.

The Joint-by-Joint Approach to Training

The joint-by-joint idea came about as a result of an off-hand conversation. Physical therapist Gray Cook and I were discussing the results we had seen in his Functional Movement Screen. I noted that difficulty in squatting always seemed to be related to limited ankle mobility. Cook's answer and subsequent analysis of the body was a straightforward one. In Cook's mind, the body is a just a stack of joints. Each joint or series of joints has a specific function and is prone to specific, predictable levels of dysfunction. As a result, each joint has specific training needs. Table 5.1 looks at the body on a joint-by-joint basis from the bottom up.

Note that the joints alternate between the need for mobility and stability as you move up the body. The ankle joint needs to be mobile, while the knee joint needs to be stable. The hip also needs to be mobile. As you follow the chain up, a simple, alternating series of joints appears.

When designing a functional workout, think about what joint the movement targets. The mobile joints need to be addressed during the warm-up sequence with rolling, stretching, and mobility work, while the stable joints are addressed during strength workouts. In essence, the joint-by-joint approach gives us targets to aim for in specific aspects of functional training.

It should be clear that injuries relate closely to proper joint function, or more appropriately to joint dysfunction. The most important concept to understand is that problems at one joint usually show up as pain in the joint above or below.

The simplest example is the lower back. It seems obvious based on the advances of the past decade that we need core stability, and it also should be obvious that many people suffer from back pain. But why do we have low back pain? Is the back weak? Stuart McGill has frequently said at seminars that people with back pain actually have stronger backs than people without back pain, so weakness is not the culprit.

In the past back pain has been blamed on a weak core. There is no strong evidence for that case, either. I believe low back pain is primarily the result of loss of

Table 5.1 Joint-By-Joint Training Needs

Joint	Need
Ankle	Mobility
Knee	Stability
Hip	Mobility
Lumbar spine	Stability
Thoracic spine	Mobility
Glenohumeral joint	Stability

hip mobility. Loss of function in the joint below (in the case of the lumbar spine, the hip) affects the joint or joints above (lumbar spine). In other words, if the hip can't move effectively, the lumbar spine will compensate. We know the hip is built for mobility and the lumbar spine is designed for stability. When the supposedly mobile joint becomes immobile, the stable joint is forced to move as compensation, becoming less stable and subsequently painful.

The process is simple: Lose ankle mobility, get knee pain. Lose hip mobility, get low back pain. Lose thoracic mobility, get neck and shoulder pain (or low back pain).

Looking at the body on a joint-by-joint basis beginning with the ankle, this thought process seems to make sense. An immobile ankle causes the stress of landing to be transferred to the joint above: the knee. In fact, I think there is a direct correlation between the stiffness of the basketball shoe and the amount of taping and bracing that correlates with the high incidence of patellofemoral syndromes in basketball players. Our desire to protect the unstable ankle comes with a high cost. Many of our athletes with knee pain have corresponding ankle mobility issues. This knee pain often follows an ankle sprain and subsequent bracing and taping.

The exception to the rule seems to be at the hip. The hip can be both immobile and unstable, resulting in knee pain from the instability (a weak hip will allow internal rotation and adduction of the femur) or back pain from the immobility. How a joint can be both immobile and unstable is the interesting question. It seems that weakness of the hip in either flexion or extension causes compensatory action at the lumbar spine, while the weakness in abduction and external rotation (or, more accurately, prevention of adduction and internal rotation) causes stress at the knee.

Poor psoas and iliacus strength or function will cause patterns of lumbar flexion as a substitute for hip flexion (see figure 5.12). Poor strength or activation of the glutes will cause a compensatory extension pattern of the lumbar spine that attempts to replace the motion of hip extension.

Interestingly enough, this fuels a vicious cycle. As the spine moves to compensate for the lack of strength and mobility of the hip, the hip loses mobility. It appears that lack of strength at the hip leads to immobility, and immobility in turn leads to compensatory motion at the spine. The end result is a kind of conundrum: a joint that needs both strength and mobility in multiple planes.

The lumbar spine is even more interesting. The lumbar spine is clearly a series of joints in need of stability, as evidenced by all the work in the area of core stability. Strangely enough, the biggest mistake I believe we have made in training over the last 10 years is engaging in an active attempt to increase the static and active range of motion of an area that obviously craves stability. I believe most if not all of the many rotary exercises done for the lumbar spine were misdirected. Both Sahrmann (2002) and

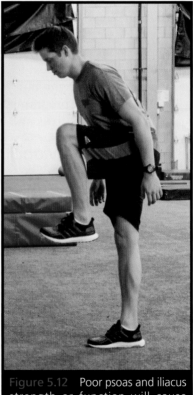

Figure 5.12   Poor psoas and iliacus strength or function will cause patterns of lumbar flexion as a substitute for hip flexion.

Porterfield and DeRosa (1998) indicate that attempting to increase range of motion in the lumbar spine is not recommended and potentially dangerous. Sahrmann states: "Rotation of the lumbar spine is more dangerous than beneficial and rotation of the pelvis and lower extremities to one side while the trunk remains stable or is rotated to the other side is particularly dangerous" (72).

I believe our lack of understanding of thoracic mobility has caused us to try to gain lumbar rotary range of motion, a huge mistake. The thoracic spine is the area we seem to know least about. Many physical therapists seem to recommend increasing thoracic mobility, and I think we will continue to see an increase in exercises designed to increase thoracic mobility. Interestingly enough, Sahrmann advocated the development of thoracic mobility and the limitation of lumbar mobility.

The glenohumeral joint is similar to the hip, meaning it is designed for mobility and therefore needs to be trained for stability. The need for stability in the glenohumeral joint presents a great case for exercises such as stability ball and BOSU ball push-ups as well as unilateral dumbbell work.

Hyman and Liponis (2005) perfectly describe our current medical system's method of reaction to injury. Icing a sore knee without examining the ankle or hip is like pulling the battery out of the smoke detector to silence it. Pain, like the sound of a smoke detector, is a warning of some other problem.

Mobility Work

The key to mobility work is that it should be done only for those joints that need it. The joints that need stability need strength training to create that stability. The joints that need mobility need motion. It is important to again mention that mobility and flexibility are not the same. Flexibility targets the muscles and tends to require some element of a static hold. Mobility targets the joints and requires gentle motion. Mobility exercises may also be viewed as activation exercises because they are designed to, as physical therapist Shirley Sahrmann likes to say, "get the right muscle moving the right joint at the right time."

Note: In four-day programs, mobility work will be done on days 2 and 4 with the lateral warm-up drills and ladder work.

Thoracic Spine Mobility

The thoracic spine is one of the least understood areas of the body and was previously the realm of physical therapists. Sue Falsone, former head athletic trainer for the Los Angeles Dodgers, may be single-handedly responsible for introducing the athletic world to the need for thoracic mobility and more importantly for showing many of us in the world of strength and conditioning a simple way to develop it. The nice thing about T-spine mobility is that almost no one has enough and it seems to be hard to get too much. We encourage our athletes to do thoracic mobility work every day.

T-SPINE DRILL 1

Our number one thoracic mobility drill is to simply foam roll the thoracic spine. As mentioned in the rolling section, it is important to touch the elbows together to protract the shoulder blades and expose the thoracic vertebrae.

T-SPINE DRILL 2

Our number two thoracic mobility drill requires just two tennis balls, so there really is no excuse. Simply tape the two balls together and go to work. The drill is basically a series of crunches beginning with the balls at the thoracolumbar junction. The balls sit over the erectors and effectively provide an anterior–posterior mobilization of the vertebrae with every little mini-crunch. It is important to return the head

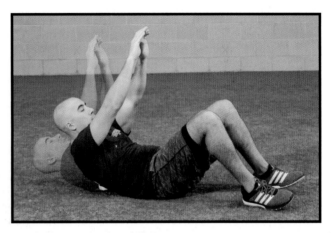
Figure 5.13   T-spine drill 2.

to the floor after every crunch and to bring the hands forward at a 45-degree angle (see figure 5.13). Do five reps at each level and simply slide down about a half roll of the ball. Work from the thoracolumbar junction up to the beginning of the cervical spine. Stay out of the cervical and lumbar areas—these areas do not need mobility work.

T-SPINE DRILL 3

The third exercise is a quadruped T-spine mobilization (see figure 5.14). This exercise adds a combination of spinal flexion, extension, and rotation to again target the thoracic spine. Begin on all fours with the butt back to the heels. One hand is placed behind the head, and the action is an elbow to elbow combination of flexion and rotation. Generally 5 to 10 reps are done on each side.

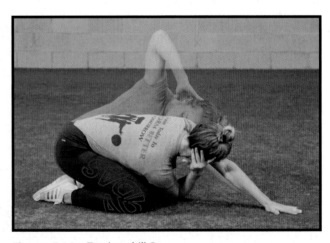
Figure 5.14   T-spine drill 3.

Ankle Mobility

Ankle mobility is step two in our warm-up. As with thoracic mobility, it is rare to find a person who doesn't need some ankle mobility work, whether you are an athlete who experienced an ankle sprain years ago (and who hasn't?) or a woman who wears heels every day.

▶ ANKLE MOBILITY DRILL 1

Credit for this drill goes to Omi Iwasaki, another EXOS physiotherapist. The first key to ankle mobility work is understanding it is a mobility drill (see figure 5.15), not a flexibility drill. You want to rock the ankle back and forth, not hold the stretch.

The second key is to watch the heel. It is essential that the heel stay in contact with the floor. Most people who have ankle mobility restrictions will immediately lift the heel. I will often hold the heel down for beginners so they get the feel of it. The third key is to make the movement multiplanar. I like 15 reps, 5 to the outside (small toe), 5 straight, and 5 driving the knee in past the big toe.

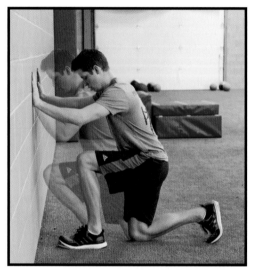

Figure 5.15   Ankle mobility drill 1.

▶ ANKLE MOBILITY DRILL 2

Leg swings. Leg swings are an interesting exercise. I used to think of leg swings as a hip mobility exercise and a dynamic adductor stretch. Physical therapist Gary Gray made me realize that leg swings are actually a great transverse-plane mobility exercise for the ankle. Yes, I said ankle. Watch an athlete with poor ankle mobility do leg swings and you will see the foot move into external rotation (turn out) with each swing. The key to leg swings is to keep the foot in contact with the floor and to drive rotary motion into the foot and ankle (see figure 5.16). The action of the leg swinging creates mobility at the ankle in the transverse plane.

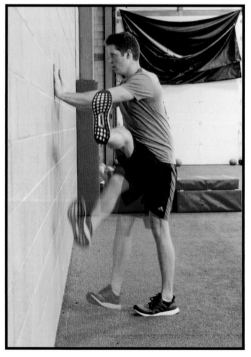

Figure 5.16   Ankle mobility drill 2.

Hip Mobility

As with thoracic and ankle mobility, it is rare to find a person who doesn't need some hip mobility work. In fact hip mobility is probably more necessary for a majority of athletes.

HIP MOBILITY DRILL 1

Split squats. Your first reaction might be that "split squats are a strength exercise." In reality, the split squat (see figure 5.17) is a sagittal-plane hip mobility exercise. To prevent soreness and develop mobility, we have our athletes perform these in place for three weeks before moving to lunges. Dan John is fond of saying, "If something is important, do it every day." This means athletes can do single-leg work every day. Some days we do split squats for mobility development, and some days we do them under load for strength. Many of the mobility exercises we use as warm-ups are the same ones we use for strength.

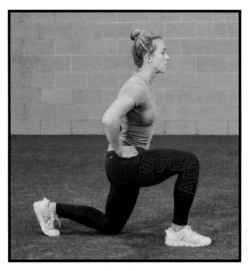

Figure 5.17   Hip mobility drill 1.

HIP MOBILITY DRILL 2

Lateral squats. Lateral squats (see figure 5.18) are the in-place precursor to lateral lunges. They develop frontal-plane hip mobility, an area where many athletes are restricted. The key in lateral squats is to watch the feet—they must remain straight ahead. External rotation is compensation. Lateral squats are a bit counterintuitive. A wider stance makes them easier, not harder, but most people try to begin narrower. Try to get the feet 3.5 to 4 feet (1 to 1.2 m) apart. I use the lines on roll flooring (usually 4-foot rolls) or the width of the wood on the lifting platforms (also usually 4 feet) as a gauge.

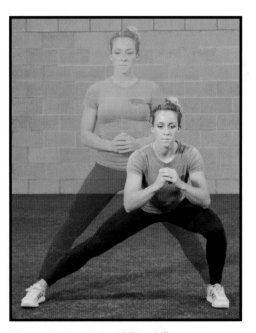

Figure 5.18   Hip mobility drill 2.

▶ HIP MOBILITY DRILL 3

Reaching single-leg straight-leg deadlift. (See figure 5.19.) As mentioned earlier, the basic patterns are done multiple times per week, sometimes under load and sometimes as warm-up and mobility work.

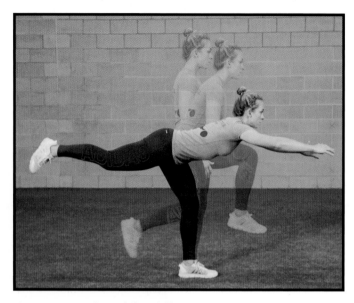

Figure 5.19   Hip mobility drill 3.

Upper Body Mobility and Stability

 Floor slides (see figure 5.20) offer multiple mobility and stability benefits for the upper body. They

- activate the low traps, rhomboids, and external rotators;
- stretch the pecs and internal rotators; and
- decrease the contributions of the upper traps.

When first trying floor slides, some athletes are surprised to find they can't even get into the position. This is not unusual. Many are also surprised by the asymmetry of their shoulders. A third surprise might occur when they try to slide overhead. Many people will immediately shrug. This is the dominance of the upper trap.

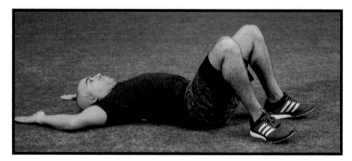

Figure 5.20   Floor slides.

Here are the keys to the floor slide:

- Retract and depress the scapulae.
- Keep the hands *and wrists* flat against the floor (ideally the backs of both hands must touch the floor).
- While sliding overhead, think about pressing gently into the floor with the forearms.
- Move only to the point of discomfort. The anterior shoulder will release and range of motion will increase. Don't force it.

DYNAMIC WARM-UP

The standing dynamic portion of the warm-up should gradually increase the stress on the muscle, get the joints moving, and activate and elongate muscles. A proper warm-up moves from rolling to stretching to mobility and activation exercises and progressively increases the intensity of the movement. The exercises should first stress flexibility and then stress movement.

A secondary benefit of a functional warm-up is that it reinforces the fundamentals of proper movement while also preparing the body to perform more intense plyometric drills, speed improvement drills, or lateral movement drills.

A good warm-up should emphasize proper foot placement in all standing drills so that while warming up, the athlete also begins to understand the relationship of foot position to force production. In simplest terms, feet put down under the hip can become accelerators. Feet put down in front of the body act as brakes. In addition, all drills should be done with perfect body position. Athletes should learn to move from the hips and not to bend at the waist.

Warm-ups and movement training can be divided into linear days and lateral days. This division, which is the brainchild of EXOS founder Mark Verstegen, is the best way to logically organize the movement portions of the workout. Linear warm-up is used to prepare the athlete for straight-ahead speed, plyometrics, and conditioning, and lateral warm-up is used to prepare the athlete for side-to-side movement, lateral plyometrics, and lateral conditioning.

Linear Active Warm-up

The linear active warm-up is simply a grouping of dynamic stretches and sprint-related drills that prepare the body for straight-ahead sprinting. Linear warm-up moves from standing dynamic stretching exercises to what most coaches would classify as form running. The form-running drills are a variation of a track-and-field dynamic warm-up. These drills are great not only for teaching movement skills but also for preparing the lower body for the speed work to follow.

Form-running drills allow an athlete to warm up the prime mover while providing a gentle dynamic stretch to the antagonist. This is what makes the linear warm-up so beneficial. Both requirements of a proper warm-up are met: The muscle temperature is raised, and the muscle is actively taken through its full range of motion. Never assume that one of these two is enough. Stretching takes the muscle through its full range, but not actively. Jogging increases muscle temperature but does not take the muscle through anything resembling full range. To properly prepare athletes for most sports, a linear warm-up must include drills that are done both forward and in reverse, so it must also include backward running

THERE'S A REASON THERE'S A BOX

How often have you heard someone described as an "out-of-the-box thinker" or heard someone praised for "thinking outside the box"? This is usually considered a compliment. However, most people would do well to really familiarize themselves with what's inside the box. I like to think that the coaches I admire achieved their success by first knowing the subject matter inside out rather than by thinking outside the box.

Coach John Wooden has a great quote: "If you spend too much time learning the tricks of the trade you may not learn the trade." He was a brilliant man, and the way he coached basketball was amazingly simple. In fact, he began every year with a detailed explanation of how to put on your socks to avoid blisters. This could be described as very inside-the-box thinking. In fact, some coaches might view something as mundane as this a waste of time. Wooden viewed players missing practice from blisters caused by not putting socks on correctly (no wrinkles inside the shoes) as the real waste of time, and he was correct. Wooden drilled fundamentals. Very inside the box.

To be honest, most of the best coaches I know talk about simplicity more than complexity. EXOS founder Mark Verstegen likes to use the phrase "simple things done savagely well" in his talks, while Dewey Nielsen of Impact Performance Training implores us to be brilliant at the basics. There is a Buddhist quote that says, "In the beginner's mind there are many choices, in the expert's mind there are few." I think there is a reason I often agree with so many of the people I consider to be good coaches. Those who have attained the expert level seem to think very much alike and react in very similar ways to new information. The experts are open to change and have great mental filters. As a result the best coaches seem to end up at the same places even when coming from different paths.

People might view me as an out-of-the-box thinker, but that may be based on 30 years in the box. The truth is I can't tell you how often I give the same answer to a different question. People ask questions and I tell them to KISS it (and I don't mean my rear end). I tell them, "Keep It Simple, Stupid." Stay in the box. Out-of-the-box thinking should be reserved for those who know the inside of the box like the literal back of their hand.

Next time you hear someone described as an out-of-the-box thinker, ask yourself if the person being referred to is also the master of the box. The key for us as coaches is to become masters of the box well before we start thinking outside of it.

---

drills. Remember, going in reverse may not matter in track and field, but it will matter in most other sports. One of the major mistakes made in teaching speed is too much reliance on information from track and field. Although most of what we know about speed comes from track and field, you need to think outside the box to apply some of these concepts to other sports.

The linear active warm-up focuses primarily on the three muscle groups most often strained in running activities: the hip flexors, hamstrings, and quadriceps. The initial six exercises are slower, dynamic stretches. The next series (skips and runs) are faster and more active to now activate what has been elongated.

Linear Active Warm-Up (20 yards or meters each)

High-knee walk

Leg cradle

Walking heel to butt

Walking heel-up to butt with forward lean

Backward lunge walk with hamstring stretch

Backward straight-leg deadlift walk

High-knee skip

High-knee run

Heel-up

Straight-leg walk

Straight-leg skip

Backpedal

Backward run

By the end of a proper linear warm-up, the muscle groups should have been taken through their full range of motion in a slow to fast sequence. This type of warm-up should precede sessions involving any type of linear movement such as sprints, plyometrics, track work, or shuttle runs. Never assume that raising muscle temperature is enough. The warm-up must prepare the muscle to move at the speed it will need to move and through the required range of motion.

HIGH-KNEE WALK

The high-knee walk is a gentle start to the warm-up that begins to stretch the muscles of the posterior hip, most importantly the glutes. When stepping forward, grasp the shin of the opposite leg and pull the knee toward the chest (see figure 5.21). Concentrate on extending the stepping leg, and get up on the toes. The action of extending the leg and rising on the toes also stretches the opposite-side hip flexor.

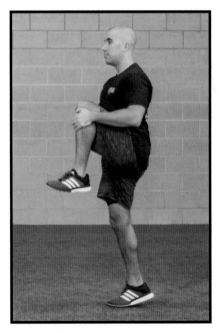

Figure 5.21   High-knee walk.

LEG CRADLE

In the leg cradle, grasp the knee with the same-side hand and the shin with the other. Hug the leg into the chest while the hand on the shin externally rotates the hip (see figure 5.22). At the same time, extend the hip of the supporting leg while rising up on the toes. Don't allow two hands on the shin. This will cause the knee to drop to waist height.

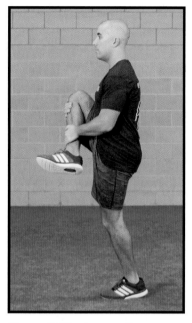

Figure 5.22   Leg cradle.

WALKING HEEL TO BUTT

Grasp the foot with the same-side hand and pull the heel to the butt with each step while walking (see figure 5.23). Once the heel is to the butt, fire the adductors and attempt to touch knee to knee. This targets the lateral quad and IT band.

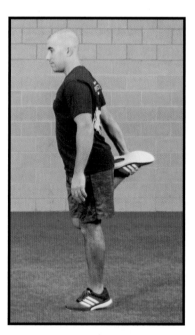

Figure 5.23   Walking heel to butt.

WALKING HEEL-UP TO BUTT WITH FORWARD LEAN

As in the previous exercise, pull the heel to the butt. In addition, lean forward, keeping the trunk straight, and lift the knee as high as possible (see figure 5.24). This exercise stresses the quadriceps and the rectus femoris of the lifted leg while also providing great proprioceptive input to the supporting foot and ankle.

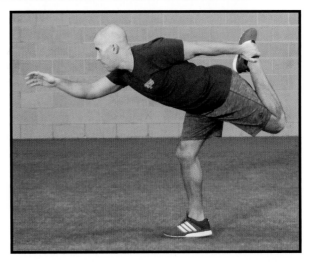

Figure 5.24   Walking heel-up to butt with forward lean.

BACKWARD LUNGE WALK WITH HAMSTRING STRETCH

This is the most technically demanding of all the exercises described. The exercise involves a combination of two backward lunges with a hamstring stretch in between (see figure 5.25). The backward lunge is a great exercise to stretch out the anterior hip while warming up all of the leg and hip extensors. It should be done with a strong overhead reach. Adding an overhead reach to the backward lunge stretches the anterior core and hip flexors simultaneously. The push-off makes this an excellent exercise for warming up the quadriceps. From the first backward lunge, place both hands on either side of the front foot and extend the front leg to create a hamstring stretch. From the hamstring stretch, return to the back lunge position and then push off and switch legs. The sequence is

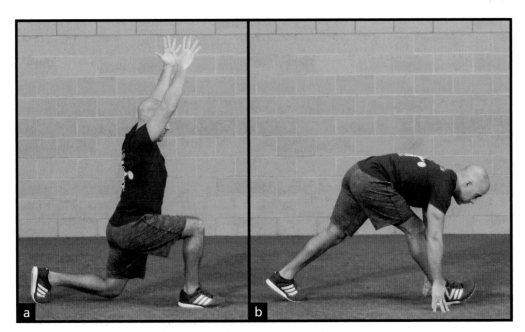

Figure 5.25   Backward lunge walk with hamstring stretch.

back lunge with overhead reach, hamstring stretch, back lunge and switch. I like to do three reps on each side to really concentrate. If you do this for distance, athletes will rush through and miss the details.

Note: Forward lunge walks place more stress on the legs than many athletes are used to, and 10 yards of forward lunge walks can leave beginners so sore that they are unable to complete the rest of the workout. Athletes who have not performed lunge walks may describe a feeling like a pulled groin muscle. Actually, this single-leg strength workout has stressed the long adductors in their function as hip extensors. This results in an unusual and unfamiliar soreness for many athletes. Generally, athletes at our training facility begin with the backward lunge walk (see figure 5.25a), as this stresses the knee extensors to a greater degree and places less stress on the long adductors.

▶ BACKWARD STRAIGHT-LEG DEADLIFT WALK

The straight-leg deadlift walk is another great active hamstring stretch. In addition, it offers excellent proprioceptive stimulus for the muscles in the ankle. Reach both arms as far forward as possible while attempting to lift one leg up to waist height (see figure 5.26). This action provides an excellent dynamic stretch of the hamstring of the supporting leg while also activating the hamstring of the opposite leg as a hip extensor. The instruction should be to "get as long as possible." I like to reinforce the visual of reaching for one end of the room or field with the hands while reaching for the other end with the foot. From this long stretch position, simply fall back one big step, landing on the opposite foot. Be careful with this exercise, as it can cause some hamstring soreness in beginners.

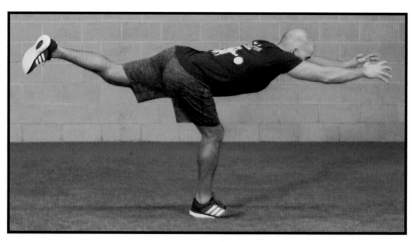

Figure 5.26   Backward straight-leg deadlift walk.

HIGH-KNEE SKIP

The high-knee skip (see figure 5.27) is the first exercise to move from dynamic stretching to a more active warm-up. The action should be gentle skipping designed to put the hip flexor and extensor musculature into action. There is no emphasis on height or speed, only on rhythmic action. The high-knee skip begins the shift toward a faster, less flexibility-oriented portion of the warm-up. With skips, think knee up, heel up, toes up. The knee should come up to waist height, the heel should come up toward the butt, and the foot should be pulled up to the shin.

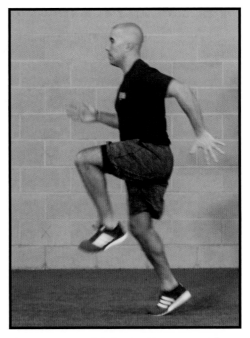

Figure 5.27   High-knee skip.

HIGH-KNEE RUN

The stress on the hip flexor group is increased in the high-knee run. This action is similar to running in place with a small degree of forward movement. Emphasis is on maintaining an upright posture (weak athletes tend to lean forward or back) and getting a large number of foot contacts. The key to this drill is to maintain perfect posture so that the stress is on the correct muscles (see figure 5.28). The best cue in the high-knee run is to have the athlete think about stepping over the height of the opposite knee. We tell our athletes to visualize a peg sticking out of the down leg at the knee. The cue is to step over the peg. Again the key is the cue of "knee up, heel up, toe up." This means the knee should be lifted to waist height, the heels pulled toward the butt, and the anterior tibialis activated to lift the toes.

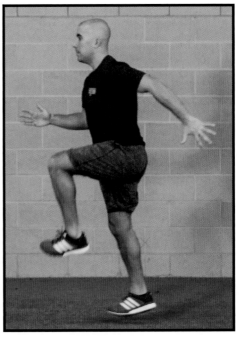

Figure 5.28   High-knee run.

HEEL-UP

The heel-up, or butt kick as it is sometimes called, shifts the emphasis from the hip flexors to the hamstrings. Actively bringing the heel to the butt not only warms up the hamstrings but also takes the quadriceps through its full range of motion. In heel-ups there can be a slight knee lift (see figure 5.29).

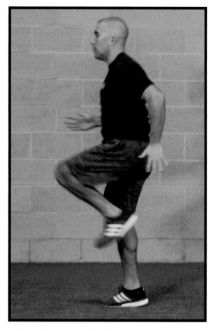

Figure 5.29   Heel-up.

STRAIGHT-LEG WALK

The straight-leg walk (figure 5.30) increases the dynamic stretch on the hamstrings while also activating the hip flexors. The hip flexors must contract powerfully to flex the hip with the leg straight. The key is to actively get the hamstrings to pull down. As mentioned later, the hamstrings are very powerful hip extensors and need to be warmed up in their extensor capacity.

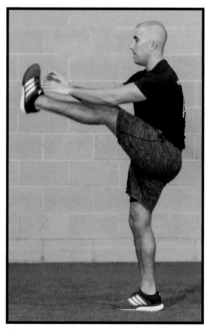

Figure 5.30   Straight-leg walk.

STRAIGHT-LEG SKIP

The straight-leg skip simply adds the rhythmic skipping action to the straight-leg walk. (figure 5.31) In addition, the dynamic stretch to the hamstring is increased by the straight-leg skipping action.

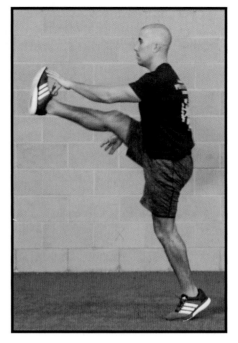

Figure 5.31   Straight-leg skip.

BACKPEDAL

It is important to clearly distinguish the backward run from the backpedal. They may appear similar, but they have completely different purposes in the warm-up sequence. The backpedal is used to warm up the quadriceps, not the hamstrings. In the backpedal, the hips are kept low, and the feet are either under the body or in front of it (see figure 5.32). The action is a quadriceps-dominant push with no reach to the rear. The feet never get behind the body as they do in the backward run. Concentrate on the extension action of the pushing leg. This is a motion that football defensive backs perform easily but that many other athletes struggle with.

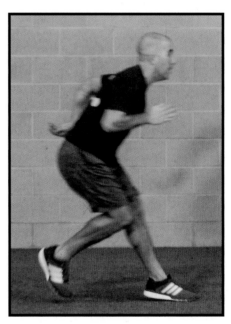

Figure 5.32   Backpedal.

BACKWARD RUN

The backward run (figure 5.33) is literally running in reverse. The emphasis is on actively pushing with the front leg while reaching out aggressively with the back leg. Backward running strongly activates the hamstrings as a hip extensor and dynamically stretches the anterior hip. This movement activates the hamstrings while stretching the hip flexors. In effect, it is the opposite of the straight-leg skip.

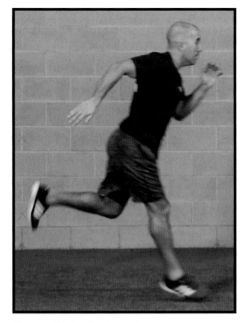

Figure 5.33   Backward run.

Developing Linear Speed Safely and Easily

Let's clear up one point: Sport is about acceleration, not speed.

We have a problem in sports. Coaches consistently use the wrong term when discussing the quality they covet most. Tests such as the 10-, 20-, and 40-yard dash are actually tests of acceleration not speed. You need only look at world-class sprinters to realize that top speed is not achieved until approximately 60 meters. As coaches our interest is not in top speed but rather in acceleration, the zero to sixty of the auto world. How rapidly an athlete accelerates will determine success in team sports, not what her absolute speed is.

Why does this matter? A great deal of the research on speed development focuses on speed in a track and field context and not in a sport context. In track the shortest event is the 55 meters. In sport the long event is a 40-yard dash (although baseball will go to 60). The track influence may in fact have limited application to sport because of sport's frequent use of acceleration mechanics versus speed mechanics. In training for track, coaches frequently make reference to the pulling action in running and work on drills to develop a pawing action against the ground. In sport the action is primarily pushing with the center of gravity slightly ahead of the feet, kind of a reverse Michael Johnson. This may mean that much of what we currently view as speed development work may have limited application to team sport athletes. In truth little can be said about speed development that has not already been said by respected coaches in their videos and lectures over the past 20 years. Information on the technical aspects of speed development is readily available from a number of different sources.

Coaches are increasingly aware that athletes need to train for strength and power to improve speed. Many coaches use resisted methods of speed development. Numerous companies provide coaches with commercial tools for speed development, such as sleds. One thing we do know is that if an athlete wants to be fast over short distances, she had better be running fast over short distances. Another thing we know is that putting force into the ground matters. There is a strong correlation between speed and vertical jump and a pretty good correlation between vertical jump and lower body strength. In a sense, getting fast is simple and hard at the same time. The concept is simple. The execution can be hard.

I propose a system of speed development, or more aptly acceleration development, with an emphasis on injury prevention for team sports and large or small groups. This system of linear speed improvement is simple and easy to implement. The majority of speed work in this system is done over less than 10 yards or meters and is actually acceleration work. Acceleration is of much greater importance in team sports than speed; however, coaches often use the words interchangeably. Coaches often express a desire for greater speed when, in fact, most sports favor athletes with greater acceleration, not necessarily the fastest athletes. The simplest analogy to describe the difference between speed and acceleration is to look at automobiles. Every car can go 60 miles per hour. What separates a Porsche from a Yugo is how fast it can get from 0 to 60. An unnecessary concern with speed rather than acceleration is the pitfall of many treadmill-oriented speed development programs and many track-and-field-based programs.

The big questions in designing a speed development program involve which drills to perform, how far to perform them, and how often to perform them. The proposed system was initially field-tested with 400 athletes in the summer of 2000 in approximately 19,000 workouts (400 athletes working out four days per week for 12 weeks) and yielded fewer than 10 groin and hamstring strains.

The keys to the system are as follows:

- Every speed workout is preceded by at least 15 minutes of dynamic warm-up and agility work.
- Plyometrics are done after warm-up and before sprinting. This seems to provide a good speed-of-contraction bridge to sprinting.

The program is broken down into three three-week phases based on simple concepts.

Weeks 1 to 3: Noncompetitive Speed

In the noncompetitive speed phase, simple drills work on the first three to five steps. Emphasis is on starting technique and first-step quickness. Athletes execute three to five hard pushes and then coast. At first, encourage them to run at slightly less than full speed to facilitate gradual muscular adaptation to sprinting. At no time should athletes race or compete in any form in this noncompetitive phase. The primary drills used in this phase are the lean, fall, and run (figure 5.34) and the 90-degree lean, fall, and run from Vern Gambetta's *Straight Ahead Speed* video (1995). Generally only six 10-yard sprints are done each day.

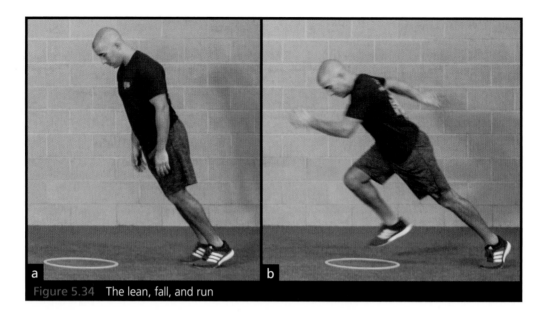

Figure 5.34 The lean, fall, and run

Weeks 4 to 6: Short Competitive Speed

The second phase introduces a series of competitive drills, but the distance is limited. The intensity of the sprint work increases while the distance (volume) is maintained. One of the difficulties of speed development programs is that coaches often cannot control or discern whether athletes are actually attempting to reach top speed during speed development sessions. The introduction of a competitive incentive ensures that athletes attempt to accelerate. The competitive incentive is simply a tennis ball. The short competitive speed phase consists of ball-drop sprints from various double- and single-leg start positions (see figure 5.35). Ball-drop sprints ensure that athletes accelerate for a short burst of speed. Even gifted athletes do not generally exceed 7 yards. Athletes frequently lay out to get the ball, although this is discouraged. Ball-drop sprints create a competitive environment that encourages acceleration without excessively stressing the hamstrings or hip flexors.

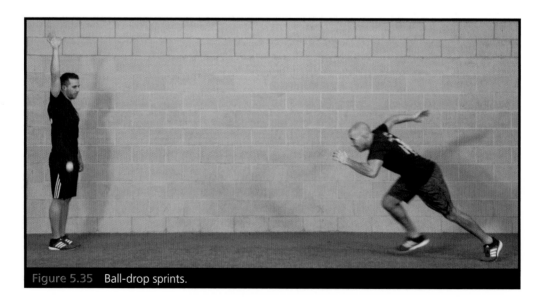

Figure 5.35 Ball-drop sprints.

Weeks 7 to 9: Long Competitive Speed

In the third phase athletes sprint against a partner from many different start positions. Chase sprints and breakaway-belt sprints are done from standing and lying starting positions. At this point, sprint workouts become tag games, with athletes alternating as the chaser or the chased. Athletes' accelerative abilities are challenged in a competitive atmosphere that guarantees maximum effort. In this phase, athletes are limited to a 10- to 20-yard tag zone.

This speed development program yields excellent results when combined with a proper warm-up, a proper lower body strength program, and a progressive plyometric program. Athletes progress gradually from individually paced starting and first-step drills to highly competitive tag races over a nine-week period to ensure proper muscular adaptation. Either volume or intensity is increased in each phase, but never both. In the lower body strength program, exercises are performed twice weekly for both knee extension (split squat versus front squat and single-leg variations) and hip extension (straight-leg and bent-leg variations that emphasize glutes and hamstrings). The combination of progressive speed, progressive plyometrics, and progressive strength training has resulted in an injury rate of less than 1 per 1,000 workouts at our training facility.

Sled Training

There is nothing better than a weighted sled to help an athlete improve his speed. In fact, if I had limited time and could do only one exercise, it might be a sled push. Numerous studies have attempted to discredit the use of a weighted sled as a tool for speed development, citing the weighted sleds' limited effect on top speed.

In truth, the evidence that weighted sleds may not improve top-speed running does not apply to acceleration and may have led coaches to undervalue a potentially valuable piece of equipment. In fact, many authors who stated that the weighted sled did not improve speed indicated that it improved acceleration. Our problem, as is often the case, was that we misinterpreted the results of the research.

Most coaches spend time working on form running and technique to improve speed. These same coaches also include lower body strength workouts to improve strength. Although these are both obviously important, there may be a missing link—the development of specific strength. How often have we seen athletes who run "pretty" but not fast? In my opinion, many coaches attempting to develop speed spend far too much time on technique drills and far too little time on developing the specific power and specific strength necessary to run faster.

In 2000 the *Journal of Applied Physiology* published an article called "Mechanical Basis of Human Running Speed." The article synopsis begins with the line "Faster top running speeds are achieved with greater ground forces, not more rapid leg movements." This has become known as the Weyland study after lead researcher Peter Weyland. Weighted sled drills target the specific muscles used in sprinting and help bridge the gap between form-running drills and weight room exercises such as squats and Olympic lifts.

Many athletes can squat large amounts of weight. Far fewer athletes seem to be able to run fast. Any student of speed will tell you that many of the strength exercises commonly recommended for speed development work hip extension but not hip hyperextension. In running speed, all of the force production is from hip hyperextension. The ability to apply force to the ground and create forward movement can occur only when the foot is placed under the center of mass and pushed back. Although squats and other exercises will train the muscles involved, the training is not specific to the act of sprinting. This may be one reason we see a higher correlation to vertical jump improvement than to speed improvement through strength training. A weighted sled teaches strong athletes how to produce the type of force that moves them forward. The sports scientists like to break this down into special strength and specific strength. Although I believe the difference is minimal, it is important to understand the difference between the two.

- Special strength is produced by movements with resistance that incorporate the joint dynamics of the skill. Sled marching would fall into the special strength category. I believe sled marching may be the best tool available for speed development. An athlete's inability to produce force in the action of sprinting becomes glaringly obvious in sled marching.
- Specific strength is produced by movements with resistance that are imitative of the joint action. I would place sled running in the specific strength category.

At MBSC we like to do sled marching with heavy loads for the first 6 weeks of a 12-week training cycle and then do 6 weeks of sled sprints with lighter loads.

In the past coaches have recommended that resisted speed development work must not slow the athlete down more than 10 percent or must not involve more than 10 percent of the athlete's body weight. These recommendations seem to be based on motor learning research indicating that excessive loads would alter the motor patterns of activities such as sprinting and throwing. I have always felt there was a missing link to speed development, but until a few years ago this so-called 10 percent rule kept me from aggressively pursuing my gut feeling. Presently, my feeling is that loads up to and exceeding the athlete's body weight can be used for special strength work as long as the athlete exhibits a motor pattern similar to the acceleration phase of sprinting. Think of sled marching as a special type of leg press. Athletes incorporate the joint dynamics of sprinting through hip hyperextension against resistance. This can be an extremely heavy movement as long as we get a technically sound march action (perfect posture).

With sled running, the approach moves toward specific strength. In sled running the loads will obviously be lighter, but I still do not follow the 10 percent rule. The main variable in sled training is not the weight on the sled but the motor pattern. If an athlete can hold an acceleration position and run without altering mechanics, then this is a specific strength exercise for sprinting. Why should we be limited by arbitrary guidelines like a 10 percent load or a 10 percent decrease in speed? Over 20 yards, 10 percent is two one-hundredths of a second. The key should be to look at the athlete's posture and motor pattern. If the athlete has to alter the mechanics to produce the desired action, then the load is too heavy. The 10 percent rule does not allow us to apply progressive resistance concepts to this form of training.

Another obvious but overlooked variable that alters the 10 percent rule is the surface being run on. Loads used on the sled need to be lighter on grass and heavier on AstroTurf. This simply relates to coefficient of friction. Less weight produces a large amount of friction as the sled moves through grass. On AstroTurf or a similar surface, the same weight would be too light. Another variable is a flat sled versus a double-runner sled. A flat sled will produce greater friction and as a result will necessitate a lighter load on the sled to get a similar effect.

The reality is that we may have misinterpreted the message when it comes to resistance training for sprints. Although research shows that sled training may not improve the athlete's ability to run at top speed, it will help the athlete get faster. Remember, sport is about acceleration, not top speed. Very few team sport athletes ever get to what track coaches like to call absolute speed mechanics. The weighted sled may be the most underrated tool for speed development because of our misinterpretation and misunderstanding of the research and terminology surrounding speed development.

Lateral Warm-up: Improving Lateral Agility and Speed

The lateral warm-up prepares the body for workouts devoted to improving lateral movement. It consists of approximately eight minutes of mobility work (see the sections on foam rolling, stretching, and mobility) followed by a laterally oriented dynamic warm-up. The last five minutes focus on agility ladder work. The key to the lateral warm-up is to stress the abductor and adductor groups to a greater degree than is possible or necessary in the linear warm-up. Most warm-ups tend to have a very linear track-and-field influence and do not get the athlete moving side to side. It is important that the warm-up be specific to the demands of the activities planned for that day. The lateral warm-up prepares the athlete for the lateral movement and lateral speed progressions to follow. The lateral dynamic warm-up emphasizes movement from side to side or in the frontal plane.

LATERAL SQUAT

Most coaches recognize the lateral squat as a groin stretch. I prefer to view the lateral squat as a dynamic flexibility exercise designed to improve the hips' range of motion in the frontal plane. Begin with the feet four feet (1.2 m) apart and sit to the right, keeping the left leg straight and the left foot flat (see figure 5.36). Sit as tall and as low as possible, keeping the weight on the right heel. Hold the bottom position for one second, and then switch to the left heel.

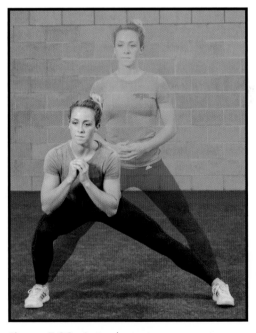

Figure 5.36   Lateral squat.

▶ LATERAL SKIP SERIES

The lateral skip series (see figure 5.37) is one of the most difficult things to teach and learn. It is best to begin with skipping in place. To lateral skip to the right, athletes must push laterally with the left leg. This introduces the idea that they move to the right by pushing with the left leg, not by stepping with the right foot. I like to teach athletes to skip in place and then think that every left contact becomes a left push. I will cue "left, left, left" as they laterally skip to their right. The action is one of abduction, or pushing out to the side.

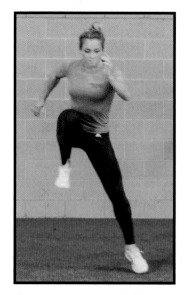

Figure 5.37 Lateral skip.

▶ CROSS-OVER SKIP

After the lateral skip is mastered, move to a cross-over skip (see figure 5.38). Now the top leg crosses over and executes the same lateral push-off. Again using the example of moving right, the left leg crosses over and comes down with a lateral push. The cueing is again a "left, left, left" sequence where the athlete focuses on the action of the left leg pushing down and across. Cross-over skipping adds a slight rotational component to the lateral movement as the knee crosses the midline of the body.

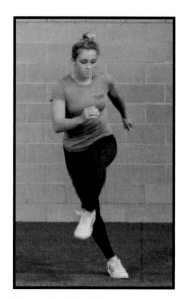

Figure 5.38 Cross-over skip.

CROSS-UNDER SKIP

The cross-under skip is identical in appearance to the cross-over but the muscle action changes. Instead of an aggressive push with the cross-over leg, the push is with the cross-under leg. This will be the most difficult of the three lateral skips for athletes to learn and in some cases will take weeks. The change here is that even though the athlete is moving to the right, the emphasis is on an aggressive lateral push with the *right* leg. The best way to grasp this mentally is to think of cross-over skip as abduction skipping, a lateral push-off using the hip abductors, and the cross-under skip as adduction skipping, a lateral push-off achieved by emphasizing the action of the under leg.

Note: In cross-over actions, both the abductors and adductors must work, and this skipping sequence begins to get athletes familiar with the qualities necessary to move laterally. It is extremely important that athletes begin to grasp the concept that a cross-over involves an abduction push of the leg that is crossing over in combination with an adduction push of the leg that is underneath.

LATERAL SHUFFLE

The lateral shuffle (see figure 5.39) is as simple as it seems. The athlete moves laterally by pushing left to go right. Emphasis is on an athletic position, feet pointed straight ahead. This is a great drill for sport-specific cues. Basketball athletes may use a palms-up defensive stance, while football players may have the hands in front in a more protective position anticipating a blocker.

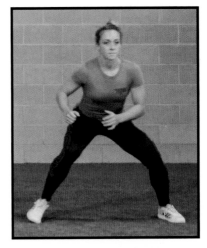

Figure 5.39   Lateral shuffle.

CARIOCA ▶

We use the standard fast-foot drill (see figure 5.40).

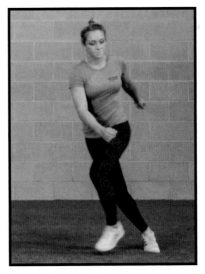

Figure 5.40   Carioca.

⏵ LATERAL CRAWL

Lateral crawling (see figure 5.41) warms up the core and scapulothoracic area from a lateral emphasis.

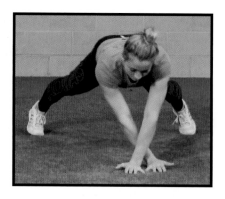

Figure 5.41   Lateral crawl.

DEVELOPING AGILITY AND DIRECTION CHANGE

The old adage that you can't teach speed was disproved years ago. However, many coaches still believe that agility and coordination cannot be taught. In truth, change of direction, the essence of lateral movement, can be taught and comes down to three simple criteria.

1. Do you have the single-leg strength necessary not only to stop movement but also to restart movement after a stop?

   Single-leg strength is the essential quality for developing agility. Without single-leg strength, no amount of agility or agility work will enable athletes to make cuts at top speed. This means single-leg work in the weight room.

2. Can you decelerate?

   Eccentric strength is the real key to deceleration. Think of eccentric strength not as the ability to lower a weight but instead as the ability to bring the body to a rapid stop. Eccentric strength is the ability to put on the brakes. This comes through plyometric drills and can also be taught with agility ladder drills.

3. Can you land with stability?

   Is the proprioceptive system prepared to create a stable landing? Again, jumps and ladder drills are key.

Athletes need to understand the most basic concept of agility: To move to the left, you must push off with the right foot. You never get anywhere fast by stepping in the direction you are going; you have to literally push yourself in the direction you want to go with the foot that is farthest away. However, before you can make the push necessary for change of direction, you need to decelerate and land with stability. Most of what passes as agility training is simply timing movement. A better philosophy is to *teach* movement, not to *time* movement. Do not just ask athletes to run around cones in an attempt to lower their time. Teach athletes the proper way to execute a right turn, a left turn, or a 45-degree cut.

To do this, we begin with simple ladder drills. Note that this piece of equipment is called an agility ladder and not a speed ladder. A ladder won't make an athlete faster, but it can improve coordination and help teach change-of-direction concepts.

QUICK FEET?

I can't tell you how often I hear someone ask, "How can I improve my son's/daughter's/athlete's foot speed or agility?" It seems that everyone always wants the shortcut and the quick fix. The better question might be "Do you think you can improve foot speed?" or maybe even the larger question "Does foot speed even matter?" This leads to "Does foot speed have anything to do with agility?"

Coaches and parents reading this are probably saying, "Is this guy crazy? How many times have we heard that speed kills?" I think the problem is that coaches and parents equate fast feet with being fast and quick feet with being agile. However, having fast feet doesn't make you fast any more than having quick feet makes you agile. In some cases fast feet might actually make you slow.

Often I see fast feet as a detriment to speed. In fact some of our quick-turnover athletes, those who would be described as having fast feet, are very slow off the start. The problem with fast feet is that you don't use the ground well to produce force. Fast feet might be good on hot coals, but they're not so great on hard ground. Think of the ground as the well from which you draw speed. It is not how fast the feet move but rather how much force goes into the ground. This is basic action–reaction physics. Force into the ground equals forward motion. This is why the athletes with the best vertical jumps are most often the fastest. It comes down to force production. Often coaches will argue that vertical jump doesn't correspond to horizontal speed, but years of data from the NFL Combine begs to differ. Force into the ground is force into the ground. The truth is parents should be asking about vertical jump improvement, not about fast feet. My standard line is "Lord of the Dance Michael Flatley has fast feet but he doesn't really go anywhere." If you move your feet fast and don't go anywhere, does it matter? It's the old "tree falling in the woods" thing.

The best solution for slow feet is to get stronger legs. Feet don't matter as much as legs matter. Think about it this way. If you stand at the starting line and take a quick first step but fail to push with the back leg, you don't go anywhere.

The reality is that a quick first step is the result of a powerful first push. We should change the buzzwords and start to say, "That kid has a great first push." Lower body strength is the real cure for slow feet and the real key to speed and agility.

I think the essence of developing quick feet lies in single-leg strength and single-leg stability work (landing skills). If you cannot decelerate you cannot accelerate, at least not more than once. One of the things I love is the magic drill idea. This is the theory that developing foot speed and agility is not a process of gaining strength and power but rather a matter of finding that perfect drill. I tell everyone I know that if I believed there was a magic drill we would do it every day. The reality is that it comes down to horsepower and the nervous system, two areas that change slowly over time.

So how do we develop speed, quickness, and agility? Unfortunately, we need to do it the slow, old-fashioned way. The key is to increase the horsepower, the brakes, and the accelerator. The answer for me is always the same—development of speed, agility, and quickness simply comes down to good training. We need to work on lower body strength and lower body power, and we need to do it on one leg.

Agility Ladder Drills

As previously mentioned, the agility ladder is a tool for warm-up, direction change, and multiplanar movement. The ladder is used for approximately five minutes twice a week and is not a cure-all or a magic drill. It is simply a great tool to teach footwork, direction change, and braking concepts as part of the warm-up. We use half ladders that are about five yards long. In addition, when choosing ladder drills I like to think about moving in all three planes. Pick at least one drill where the athlete moves across the ladder in the frontal plane, a drill where she faces the ladder and moves sagittally, and a drill with a rotary or transverse component. Remember the ladder is not a conditioning tool, and long ladders and short reps are the road to slow feet, not faster.

▶ SHUFFLE WIDE AND STICK

Popularly known as the Ickey Shuffle after Cincinnati Bengals running back Ickey Woods' touchdown dance, the shuffle wide and stick (see figure 5.42) is a three-count drill. Ladder drills break down into two-count drills with a 1-2 cadence, three-count drills with a 1-2-3 cadence, and four-count drills.

The action is in-in-out. In other words, the athlete begins on the left side of the ladder standing on the left foot. The action of the drill is now right-left-right: two feet into the ladder followed by a stable landing on the opposite side on the right foot. He wants to stick that landing for a count of one one thousand. The essence of this drill is the stutter step, which is the basic component of most offensive evasive maneuvers in sport. The cross-over dribble in basketball and the wide dribble in field or ice hockey are just a few examples of executing a stutter step to elude an opponent.

The feet should move quickly, accurately, and low to the ladder. We like to cue "in-in-out" and "stick it." The key here is fast in the ladder and a stable landing on one foot outside. With our agility ladder drills, all drills that begin facing forward are done backward on the return, so the athlete would shuffle wide and stick going forward and return in reverse. Remember, in most sports movement isn't only forward.

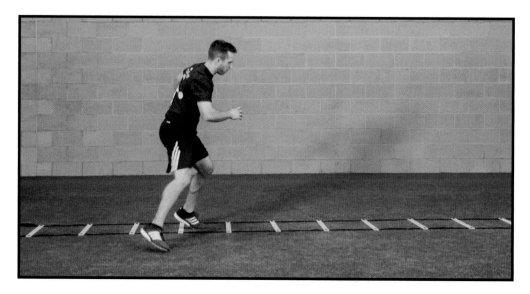

Figure 5.42   Shuffle wide and stick.

SHUFFLE QUICK

The shuffle quick is the same drill minus the stick. Instead of landing stable on the outside foot, use a quick foot action to immediately cross to the other side.

SHUFFLE QUICK AND STICK

After three weeks of learning the shuffle wide and stick and the shuffle quick, progress to sticking on one side and quick on the other (see figure 5.43). This entire sequence takes two trips up and down the ladder. Go up the ladder going quick on the right and sticking the left, coming back in reverse. Then switch sides and go quick left and stick right, both forward and backward. This is a great drill to combine the feet and the brain. The athlete has to move the feet and think, which might be the essence of sport.

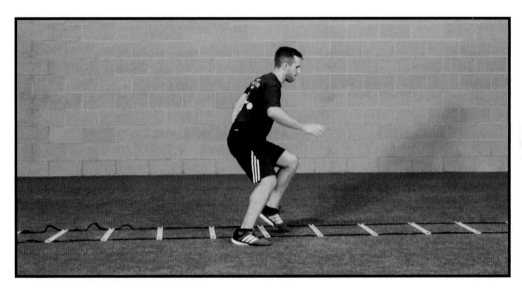

Figure 5.43   Shuffle quick and stick.

▶ CROSS IN FRONT

This is another basic three-count, quick-foot ladder drill (see figure 5.44). The sequence now is in-out-out. The athlete begins on two feet outside the ladder. From the left side, the first step is a cross-over step into the ladder with the left leg. The right then steps across the ladder, followed by the left. The sequence is left-right-left. I like to cue "cross in, out, out" so the athletes can get the thought and rhythm. I also like to use a Waltz tempo of 1-2-3, 1-2-3 to get athletes to think about foot contacts. Go up forward and back backward.

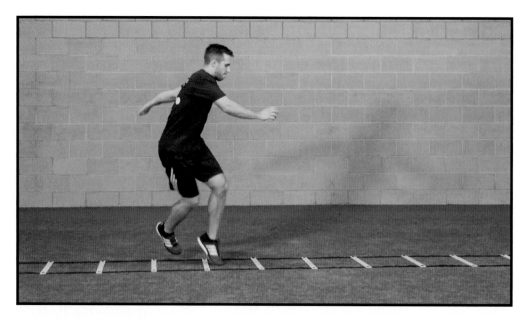

Figure 5.44   Cross in front.

HARD CROSS-OVER

This is the same foot action as the cross in front, but it is much more aggressive. Where the previous drill is a quick-foot drill, this one is a real change-of-direction drill. In the hard cross-over we cue a really aggressive push-off with the inside leg, really encouraging the athlete to lean into the ladder. The landing is a very aggressive stop in a two-foot base position, so rather than a 1-2-3 rhythm it is more of a two-count drill. The action is lean into the ladder, push hard with the inside leg to cross into the ladder, and land solid on two feet on the opposite side. The landing should mimic a skater's stop or the action of a two-foot baseball slide.

CROSS BEHIND

This is the same drill as the cross in front but the foot is now crossed behind. Many athletes struggle because this is not a common action, but teaching athletes how to get tangled up in their own feet and keep moving is valuable. In addition, in sports such as soccer and hockey, passes are often behind and can be fielded with a back-foot, cross-behind action.

IN-IN-OUT-OUT

In-in-out-out is one of my favorite drills because it can be done forward (see figure 5.45a), backward, moving right, and moving left (see figure 5.45b). This is a four-count drill that proceeds exactly as it sounds. In the forward version the athlete begins with feet straddling the ladder and moves forward by going in-in-out-out. The two feet outside the ladder move into and out of the boxes as the athlete moves forward. Right and left are done the same, but the athlete starts facing the ladder rather than straddling it.

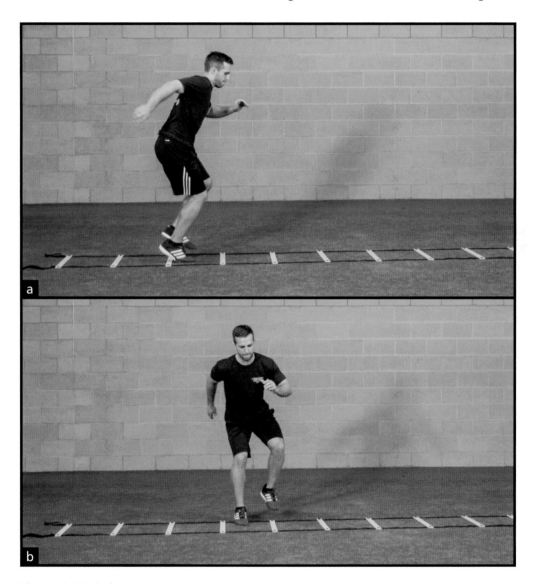

Figure 5.45   In-in-out-out.

OUT-OUT-IN-IN

I love this drill because it is more of a spatial awareness drill. The athlete begins sideways in the ladder but now must go right or left moving out of the ladder (see figure 5.46). Although this seems simple, the reversal of the position of the ladder drastically increases the difficulty.

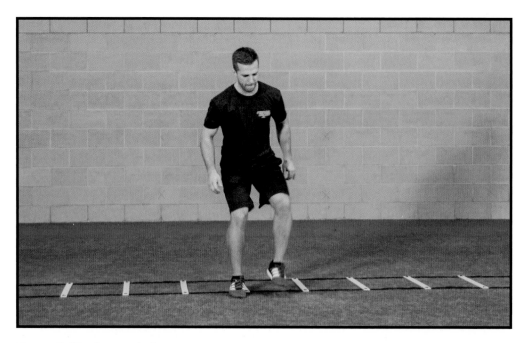

Figure 5.46   Out-out-in-in.

SCISSORS ▶

The scissors drill (see figure 5.47) is a simple lateral, sagittal-plane drill in which the athlete begins with one foot in the ladder and moves laterally by simply alternating feet. If going to the right, the athlete begins with the right foot in the first box and simply moves down the ladder in a left-right-left-right sequence.

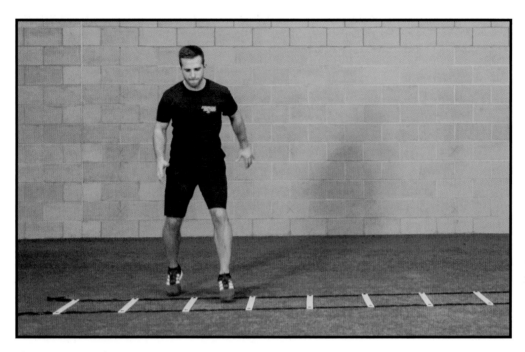

Figure 5.47   Scissors.

▶ HIP SWITCH

Hip switch (see figure 5.48) is basically scissors with a cross-over. As the feet switch, the far foot crosses over to the next box. This drill adds a rotary, or transverse, component to a lateral drill.

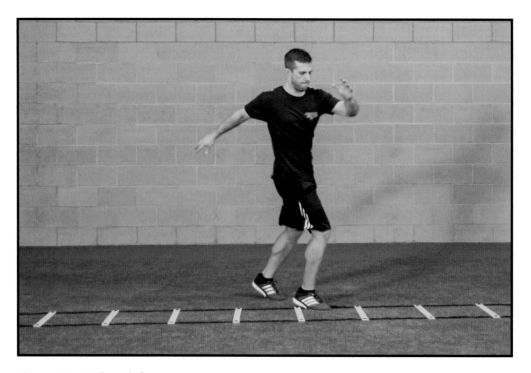

Figure 5.48   Hip switch.

There are numerous other drills to choose from with infinite variations. The key is to keep it simple. Use a mix of linear and lateral ladder drills, and include some that add a rotary component. See the ladder for what it is—a great tool for warm-up and a great tool for footwork and direction change.

This chapter provides some simple yet effective progressions to improve both linear speed and lateral movement. The athlete moves through a specific warm-up designed around drills that are appropriate for the movement emphasis of the day. Specific days are devoted to linear speed, and others are devoted to lateral movement. This simple system allows coaches to design workouts easily and athletes to be properly prepared for the stresses to follow. The warm-ups incorporate progressions for the neuromuscular system and are based on current science on warm-ups and injury reduction to ensure a safe approach. Remember, functional training is training that makes sense. A warm-up that relates to the drills and activities about to be performed also makes sense.

REFERENCES

Currier, D.P., and R.M. Nelson. 1992. *Dynamics of Human Biologic Tissues*. Philadelphia: Davis.

Davies, C., and A. Davies. 2004. *The Trigger Point Therapy Workbook*. New Harbinger Publications.

Gambetta, V. 1995. *Straight Ahead Speed* (video). Gambetta Sports Systems.

Hyman, M., and M. Liponis. 2005. *Ultra-Prevention*. Atria Books.

McGill, S.M., and S. Brown. 1992. Creep response of the lumbar spine to prolonged full flexion. *Clinical Biomechanics*. 7: 43-46.

Myers, T. 2009. *Anatomy Trains: Myofascial Meridians for Movement Therapists*. 2nd ed. Philadelphia: Churchill Livingstone, Elsevier.

Porterfield, J., and C. DeRosa. 1998. *Mechanical Low Back Pain: Perspectives in Functional Anatomy*. Philadelphia: Saunders.

Sahrmann, S. 2002. *Diagnosis and Treatment of Movement Impairment Syndromes*. St. Louis: Mosby.

Weyland, P. 2000. Mechanical basis of human running speed. *Journal of Applied Physiology*. 89(5): 1991-1999.

Wilhelmi, B.J., S.J. Blackwell, J.S. Mancoll, and L.G. Phillips. 1998. Creep vs. stretch: A review of viscoelastic properties of skin. *Annals of Plastic Surgery*. 41: 215-219.

Lower Body Training

My views on lower body training have changed drastically since the publication of the first edition of *Functional Training for Sports*. Over the past decade we have moved from a very conventional back squat oriented program to a front squat oriented program and finally to a program centered primarily around unilateral deadlifts and unilateral squat variations. In certain situations we initially use bilateral squats and bilateral deadlifts, but the emphasis has clearly moved to more unilateral exercises when it comes to developing lower body strength.

The primary reason for this evolution in lower body training strategy is our desire to most effectively achieve these three goals:

- *No injuries in training.* Almost all our athletes' back pain issues resulted from performing heavy squats.
- *Decreased injuries in the competitive season.* A program of unilateral exercises seems to have greater injury reduction benefits when compared with a program that emphasizes bilateral work.
- *Improved performance.* Athletes' using unilateral training exercises saw the same or better performance gains as when they used bilateral exercises.

Although we can agree that functional lower body strength should be the primary emphasis in any high-quality training program, many will disagree on how to develop it. We do know that nearly every team sport, and many individual sports, relies heavily on speed, and the first step in speed improvement is strength improvement. Whether the goal is performance enhancement, injury prevention, strength gains, or size gains, training the lower body is the best way to accomplish all of these.

STARTING WITH BODY-WEIGHT SQUATS

Our lower body strength training often begins with learning to body-weight squat and to do a kettlebell sumo deadlift, both bilateral exercises. The squat and hinge are still considered fundamental movement skills. However, for many athletes more hip-dominant exercises such as kettlebell sumo deadlifts or trap-bar deadlifts are a better starting point than squatting. In fact, deadlifts can be easier to learn and are often less limited by mobility issues. Teaching an athlete to perform a body-weight squat is still important, however, and will reveal important information about flexibility and injury potential.

The question now is how and whether to load the squat. Squatting and squatting under load present unique problems from both a physical and psychological standpoint. In the simplest sense we need to ask ourselves, "Should we place external load on an athlete who cannot properly perform a perfect body-weight squat?"

To understand the challenges of teaching squatting, it is critical to first examine the psychology of lifting weights in general. There is a macho aspect, most evident with young males, that makes learning strength training exercises very difficult. This motor learning process becomes particularly difficult in a group setting. Very few athletes want to go through the motion of squatting without weight to develop the mobility necessary to squat properly. Instead, athletes want to lift weights and want to be challenged.

All too often an athlete who squats poorly is still encouraged by a well-meaning coach to "get strong." Physical therapist Gray Cook describes this mistake as "adding strength to dysfunction." What Cook is saying in the simplest sense is that if you can't squat well, don't squat with weight. If we allow an athlete with poor technique to squat under load, we are simply adding strength on top of movement dysfunction. The athlete or client still has a poor pattern, but the poor pattern can now be demonstrated with an external load. This is a common high school and college strength training mistake and may be at the root of many athletes' back pain.

So instead, the initial advice a coach should give the athlete is to "get mobile" or "perfect your squat pattern." Only after the correct technique is established should an athlete add load to the lift.

Our current approach is to work on mobility to develop the squat pattern before we load it and to do the majority of our lower body squat pattern loading in unilateral exercises. The unilateral knee-dominant pattern is a simpler one to teach and is much more usable.

The bilateral squat is probably best learned as part of warm-up, assuming the warm-up is performed outside of the weight room so the athlete is not thinking, *How much weight is on the bar and who is looking at me?* From a psychological standpoint we have removed one barrier to success in learning to squat. The desire to continually add external load in the weight room forces the athlete back to faulty and familiar movement patterns. Working on squat mobility as part of warm-up does the opposite. Although we work on squat mobility in our warm-ups we simultaneously work on single-leg strength in the strength program through our unilateral lower body progressions.

Our athletes can also develop hip and back strength with exercises such as kettlebell sumo deadlifts or trap-bar deadlifts (a much simpler exercise to learn than the squat because of the decreased hip range of motion) while simultaneously working on single-leg strength and mobility.

DISTINGUISHING THE SQUAT AND DEADLIFT

When people ask me to define the difference between a squat and a deadlift I used to be able to give a simple answer. In the deadlift the weight is in the hands (see figure 6.1a). To me, that was the easiest way to distinguish between squats and deadlifts. For squats the bar is on the shoulders (see figure 6.1b), either front or back. Both lifts look a lot alike. But if a deadlift is defined by a weight in the hands, what is depicted in figure 6.2?

Readers familiar with the exercise would say that's a rear-foot-elevated split squat, or if you like silly names, a Bulgarian lunge (silly because it is neither Bulgarian nor a lunge). But isn't the weight in the hands? The argument will be that it's a squat because the torso is more erect.

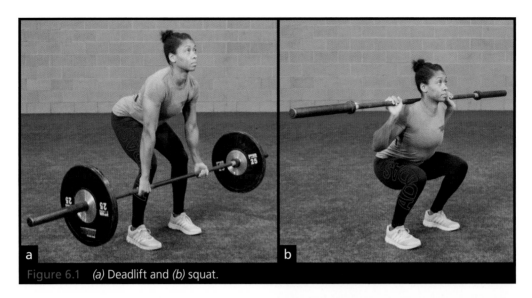

Figure 6.1   *(a)* Deadlift and *(b)* squat.

Lower body strength training can be broken down into knee-dominant patterns and hip-dominant patterns. In the old days, this broke down into bilateral squats and bilateral deadlifts and their variations.

My point is that the picture we have now is much more complicated. Our exercise menu has evolved so much that the old definitions of squat and deadlift no longer apply, and we need new ones. In the goblet squat, the weight is in the hands but above the waist. It's a squat. Maybe a type of front squat but a squat nonetheless. In the kettlebell sumo deadlift, the weight is in the hands but

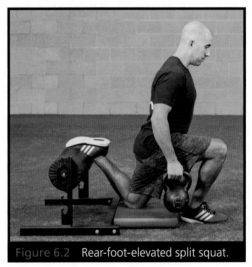

Figure 6.2   Rear-foot-elevated split squat.

the lower body pattern can be turned into a knee-dominant one that looks more like a squat than a deadlift.

Is figure 6.3 a trap-bar deadlift or trap-bar squat, or does that depend on how the exercise is done? If an exercise that is called a trap-bar deadlift has a squatting-type lower body pattern, does it then become a trap-bar squat? In a suitcase-style rear-foot-elevated split squat the weight is in the hands and below the waist, but these clearly don't seem like deadlifts.

So then we come back to the definition of a deadlift. Is it a deadlift if the weight is picked up from the ground and then brought back to the ground? That might have been my definition until I read Dan John and Pavel Tsatsouline's *Easy Strength*. The authors may have redefined squats and deadlifts. They make the distinction of a deadlift having "deep hip movement with minimal knee bend" and a squat having "deep movement of the knees *and* hips" (179).

In other words a hip-dominant movement is a deadlift and a knee-dominant movement is a squat. A hip-dominant movement has, as John and Tsatsouline say, "deep hip movement with minimal knee bend." Think kettlebell swings (see figure 6.4) and the misnamed straight-leg deadlift (see figure 6.5). I like the term *modified straight-leg deadlift*. With the popularity of swings and the emergence of the trap bar, the landscape has changed quite a bit.

Perhaps we should reexamine some exercises and classify them using John and Tsatsouline's definitions.

Let's analyze the sumo deadlift (see figure 6.6). Anterior chain? Maybe. Posterior chain? Maybe. Adductor target? Definitely. Is this a deadlift? When I was a powerlifter this was *the* deadlift for squatters. In my powerlifting days I was a sumo-style deadlifter because my legs were much stronger than my back.

A wide-stance squatter who is more anterior-chain dominant will probably pull more in the sumo deadlift than the conventional deadlift. Such a lifter basically squats the deadlift while holding the bar in the hands. In terms of knee dominant or hip dominant, I think we have to vote for knee. In the first edition of *Functional Training for Sports* I called these hybrids, exercises that didn't seem to fit neatly into the knee- or the hip-dominant categories.

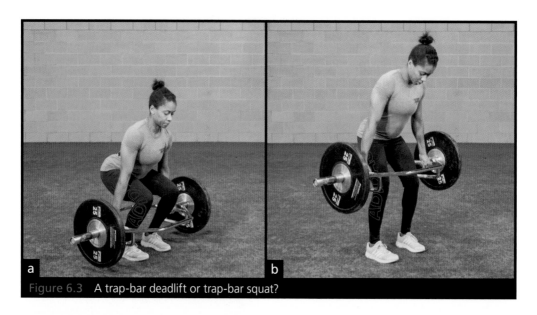

a   b

Figure 6.3　A trap-bar deadlift or trap-bar squat?

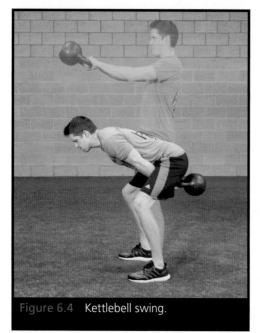

Figure 6.4　Kettlebell swing.

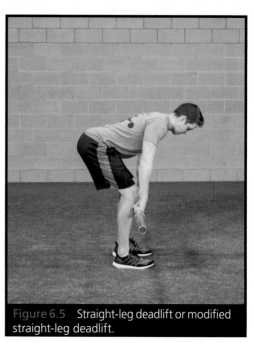

Figure 6.5　Straight-leg deadlift or modified straight-leg deadlift.

In figure 6.7*a*, the unloaded version would be a sumo squat. Add a kettlebell as indicated and it becomes a sumo deadlift (figure 6.7*b*). Move the load up to goblet position and it becomes a goblet squat (figure 6.7*c*). Confused? I hope not. The point is that things are never as clear or as simple as we would like them to be.

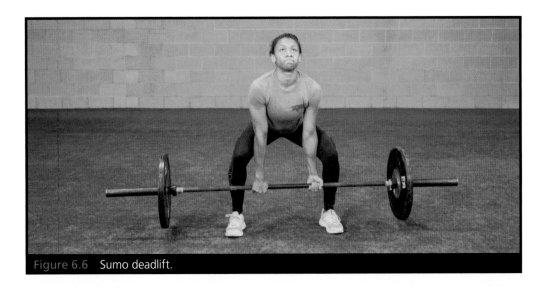

Figure 6.6   Sumo deadlift.

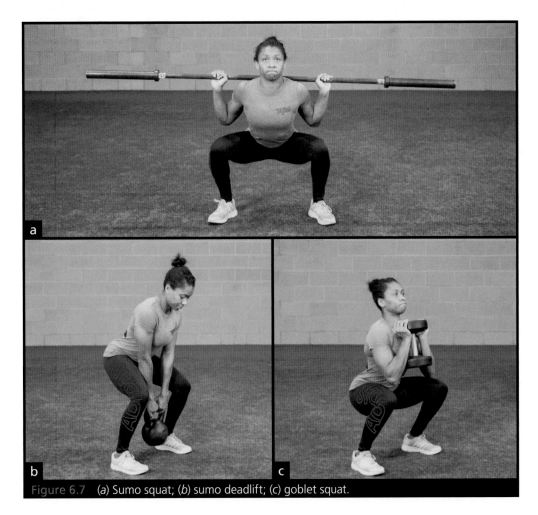

Figure 6.7   (*a*) Sumo squat; (*b*) sumo deadlift; (*c*) goblet squat.

Bottom line: Who cares? It really is just semantics. In a powerlifting meet, the deadlift will always be the lift picked up from the floor. However in gyms and sport performance programs the menu has changed. Hip hinge with minimal knee movement? Deadlift. Shared knee and hip movement? Squat.

To make matters worse (or better), I want you to teach your athletes to squat, but when they start to get strong, to switch to unilateral variations of the squat or to the trap-bar deadlift if you really want a bilateral exercise. The concept of relying primarily on unilateral training for the lower body is based on one simple thought (we run and jump on one leg most of the time) and one not-so-simple thought, something known as the bilateral deficit.

"The bilateral limb deficit (BLD) phenomenon is the difference in maximal or near maximal force generating capacity of muscles when they are contracted alone or in combination with the contralateral muscles. A deficit occurs when the summed unilateral force is greater than the bilateral force. The BLD has been observed by a number of researchers in both upper and lower limbs, in isometric and in dynamic contractions" (Kuruganti, Murphy, and Pardy 2010)

What does this mean? It means an athlete on one leg is able to squat more than half of what he can squat on two legs. We are actually stronger with one foot on the ground than we are with two feet on the ground, if you divide by two. Every athlete we train can do a rear-foot-elevated split squat with significantly more than half of what they can do in a back squat. In fact when we tested both front squats and rear-foot-elevated split squats, many of our athletes could split-squat and front-squat with the same loads. I know it seems impossible, but it's not.

So step one is still teaching the squat pattern. Notice I said *squat pattern* and not *squat*. The goal is mobility in the squat position, not getting a bar in the back or front squat position. Simply attempting to teach an athlete the body-weight squat, goblet squat, or kettlebell deadlift can reveal important information about strength, flexibility, and injury potential. Body-weight squats and goblet squats can be used to assess mobility in the hips and ankles, flexibility in the hamstrings, and the general status of the lower body.

Athletes who cannot body-weight squat to a position with the thighs parallel to the floor (see figure 6.8) tend to be deficient in ankle or hip mobility, hamstring

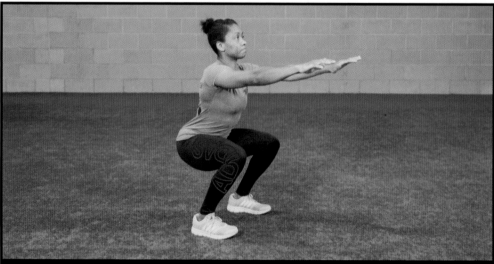

Figure 6.8   Athletes who cannot body-weight squat to a position with the thighs parallel to the floor tend to be deficient in ankle or hip mobility, hamstring flexibility, or a combination of the three.

flexibility, or a combination of the three. The first step in correcting a problem with the squat pattern is to attempt a squat with the heels elevated. Raising the heels on a one- by four-inch (2.5 by 10 cm) board or a specially made wedge should enable most athletes to squat to the proper depth. The board simply provides artificial ankle mobility.

Note: Raising the heels does not harm the knees in any way. The idea that elevating the heels increases the stress on the knees is not supported by any scientific research we have ever seen. In fact, Olympic weightlifters and competitive powerlifters have used heeled shoes in both competition and training for decades.

Proper squat patterning involves teaching the athlete to keep the weight on the heels and to sit back into the squat. When most athletes hear the directive "squat," their minds tell their bodies to lower their hips the easiest way possible.

For weaker athletes the easiest way is often one that does not overstress the weak muscles (usually the quadriceps). Weaker athletes or athletes returning from injury often attempt to lower the center of gravity by initially driving the knees forward out over the toes until the limit of the ankle range of motion is reached (see figure 6.9). Then and only then does the movement begin to center on the knee joint. This type of ankle-dominant squatting leads to excessive knee flexion in order to reach a position with the thighs parallel to the ground.

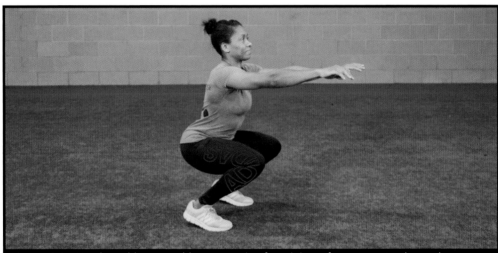

Figure 6.9   Weaker athletes or athletes returning from injury often attempt to lower the center of gravity by initially driving the knees forward out over the toes until the limit of the ankle range of motion is reached.

SQUATTING TO POWERLIFTING PARALLEL

Most therapists and athletic trainers make the mistake of describing squatting solely based on knee angle, with patients often instructed to squat to 90 degrees. However, the goal is a position where the femurs (thighbones) are parallel to the floor. A knee angle of 90 degrees can be reached far before a thighs-parallel squat is reached.

Strength coaches on the other hand do not usually define squat depth by knee angle but rather by this parallel relationship of the femurs to the floor. Squatting to a femurs-parallel position often results in a knee angle greater than 135 degrees if the athlete is an ankle-dominant squatter. This type of ankle-dominant squatting is frequently seen in athletes with knee pain or patellar tendinitis (tendinitis in the quadriceps tendon).

The key to teaching and learning the squat pattern is to combine a therapist's desire to limit the athlete's knee flexion range of motion with a coach's desire to get the athlete's thighs parallel to the floor. Coaches, trainers, and therapists need to speak the same language. The athlete must be given instructions that address both the coach's concerns and the trainer's or therapist's concerns. The athlete must be taught to perform a body-weight squat in a manner that minimizes range of motion at the ankle and maximizes range of motion at the knee.

Full-depth squatting is always taught in our program. We define a full squat as the tops of the thighs being parallel to the floor.

We have taken to using 12-inch (30 cm) plyometric boxes as depth gauges for teaching squatting. We adjust height with Airex pads to get a parallel depth, but you will be surprised by how many athletes can use a 12-inch box.

Please note these are not box squats but body-weight or goblet squats done to the box to gauge depth. Half squats or quarter squats should never be used or taught. The half squats and quarter squats often seen in poorly designed strength and conditioning programs present a larger risk of back injury due to the heavier weights used in these partial movements.

Athletes with normal flexibility can squat to a position with the thighs parallel to the floor with no heel elevation. Less flexible athletes can use heel elevation. Learning the squat pattern is the first step in increasing lower body strength, speed, and vertical jump.

The concept of squatting below parallel has become popular in some circles. However, caution should be used below the depth I would call "powerlifting parallel." Carl Klein, in his landmark work of the 1970s, *The Knee in Sports*, cautioned against performing full squats. Sadly, many read Klein's comments but not his book. As they say, the devil is in the details. Klein cautioned against full squatting and started a significant controversy. However, very few doctors who picked up on Klein's advice actually read the book or looked at the pictures.

Klein cautioned that "as full flexion is approached the anterior fibers of both the medial and lateral collateral ligaments are tightened and stretch beyond the state of their normal length. The anterior cruciate is also stretched in full knee flexion as the knee is forced apart by the fulcrum effect especially if the bulky posterior thigh and calf muscle is present. Continuous action of this nature will eventually weaken the integrity of these supporting ligaments and possibly decrease 'stretch-effect readiness' (proprioceptive stimulus) in calling for muscle support in stretch situations" (14).

Klein goes on to say that "the depth of the squat should be controlled, with the thighs just breaking the parallel position. Much beyond this point, the reaction between the hamstrings and the calf muscle begins to act as a pry to force the joint apart at the front as well as on the sides, stretching the ligaments" (30).

Even forty years later it's tough to argue with Klein's logic. There are some legitimate injury concerns with squatting to below parallel.

The major problem was in Klein's definition of a full squat. Klein's full squat was a below-parallel version used primarily by Olympic weightlifters but now popular with some of the hard-core strength crowd.

Klein brings up a very valid concern that "in the full squat position the posterior horn or rim of the medial cartilage is locked between the tibia and the femur. . . if any disruption of the mechanics of the joint takes place at this time, when the posterior part of the cartilage remains fixed and the anterior part is moving forward, a posterior tear results" (56).

The key is that "it is possible to develop great leg strength without taking the risk of bending the legs past parallel. Therefore, unless you are a competitive weightlifter who has found the squat style especially efficient you will be well advised not to squat below the parallel when exercising" (57).

Bottom line: Keep squats to "powerlifting parallel" and avoid the currently fashionable pistol-style squats.

BASELINE, REGRESSIONS, AND PROGRESSIONS

We classify our upper and lower body exercises as baseline, regressions, or progressions. Baseline exercises are the general starting point for the average athlete. From here, the athlete either progresses or regresses. Progressions are numbered in order from easy to difficult. Regressions are also numbered, but think easy, easier, easiest. Therefore progression 3 will be a fairly difficult exercise, while regression 3 will be very simple.

BODY-WEIGHT SQUAT

BASELINE

For the body-weight squat (see figure 6.10), start with the arms extended out in front of the body with the hands at shoulder height. The chest should be up, and the upper and lower back should be slightly arched and tight. Feet should be approximately shoulder-width apart and slightly turned out, approximately 10 to 15 degrees. The stance may be widened to obtain proper depth if flexibility is a problem. A one-by-four-inch (2.5 by 10 cm) board, a 10-pound (5 kg) plate, or a specially made wedge may be placed under the heels if the athlete tends to lean forward during the descent, if the heels lose contact with the ground, or if the pelvis rotates posteriorly in the descent. Although

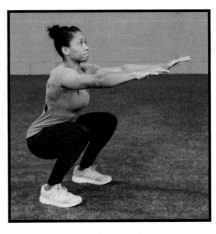

Figure 6.10   Body-weight squat.

many authorities caution against an object under the heels, athletes at our training facility have experienced great success and no knee pain with this method.

The Descent

1. Before descending into the squat, inhale deeply through the nose.
2. When descending into the squat, concentrate on sitting back and placing the body weight on the heels. I like to cue beginners to pull the toes up to the tops of the shoes. Placing the body weight on the midfoot or toes causes an undesirable forward lean. Do not let the breath out. Keep the hands level with the shoulders.
3. Descend slowly until the tops of the thighs are parallel to the floor.
4. In the descent, the knees should stay over the toes. Do not pinch the knees in; allow the knees to spread outward over the toes.

The Ascent

1. Concentrate on driving upward with the chest out, bringing the hips up and forward.
2. Drive the heels into the floor.
3. Exhale by blowing out forcefully through pursed lips as if blowing out candles.

LEARNING THE GOBLET SQUAT
REGRESSION 1 + PROGRESSION 1

The first regression in squatting involves adding weight. Surprisingly, so does the first progression. In fact the progression and regressions are the same exercise. I know this sounds contradictory, but bear with me.

GOBLET SQUAT
REGRESSION 1

At only one other point in this book do I advocate adding weight to make an exercise easier (more on this later). In fact, I know this is counterintuitive advice. I will go as far as to say that 90 percent of the time, technique problems stem from using too much weight. Learning to body-weight squat is one of the exceptions.

The first correction for any less-than-perfect squat is always a heel board or wedge as mentioned already. The second correction is to add a dumbbell in the goblet position.

In the goblet position (see figure 6.11), popularized by strength and conditioning guru Dan John, the dumbbell is held upside down by one end. John likens it to holding a large beverage goblet or bowl of soup (note: *soup bowl squats* is not nearly as catchy a term). The key is that

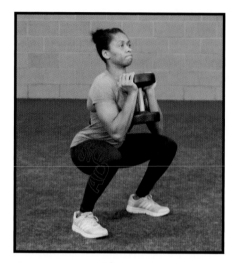

Figure 6.11   Goblet squat.

the top of the dumbbell is touching the sternum and collarbone while the bottom stays in contact with the lower sternum, or xiphoid process.

The effect of the goblet load is nothing short of miraculous. Holding a dumbbell in the goblet position can instantly turn a bad squat into a good squat. It is nothing short of magic.

After hearing Dan John sing the praises of the goblet squat over and over, we conducted a simple experiment at MBSC. We took all our bad squatters, mostly teenage boys, and added 10 to 20 pounds (5 to 10 kg) in the goblet position. The results were 100 percent favorable. Every athlete looked better. The goblet seems to serve as a reactive tool to turn on the core and upper body stabilizers. This results in a significant improvement in technique. Again, the key to goblet squats is keeping two contact points (collarbone and xiphoid) throughout the lift. If the lower contact point is lost, this indicates an undesirable forward lean that must be corrected.

Important note: Every lower body exercise that can be goblet loaded should be goblet loaded first. Use the goblet position until the athlete can no longer get the dumbbell into place. Use dumbbells instead of kettlebells to get good contact points.

GOBLET SQUAT
PROGRESSION 1

Not surprisingly, the same technique that turns a bad squat good also makes a good squat better. Our first loading option is the same for someone with perfect technique as it for someone with poor technique—add a dumbbell in the goblet position. This is the only way we load a squat until the athlete is not able to maintain the two contact points. It is not unusual for our male high school athletes to use 120-pound (55 kg) dumbbells in the goblet position. Our females easily get in the 70 to 80 pound (30 to 35 kg) range. In fact, the only time we squat with a bar is to help our athletes with Olympic lifts (more on this in chapter 10).

KETTLEBELL SUMO DEADLIFT
REGRESSION 2

I know, more confusion. First I say that if you can't squat well, try adding weight. Very counterintuitive. Now I'm saying to regress to a deadlift? I have really fallen in love with single kettlebell and single dumbbell sumo deadlifts. If you don't have kettlebells (which have convenient handles), the athlete can just flip the dumbbell upside down, place it on the floor, and grab the end. The nice thing about a kettlebell sumo deadlift is that it couldn't be simpler.

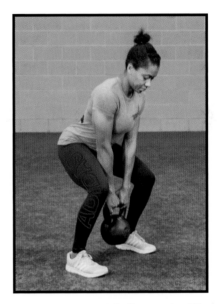

Take a squat stance, drop the butt down until the dumbbell end or the kettlebell handle is within reach, grab it, squeeze the lats and low traps, and pick it up (see figure 6.12). Some lifters will use a little more of the deadlift pattern (more hip movement, less knee movement), but that's fine.

In our experience the last few years, this has been a key regression. We continue with kettlebell or dumbbell sumo deadlifts as our primary lower body exercise until the athlete can handle the heaviest dumbbell.

Figure 6.12   Kettlebell sumo deadlift.

Note: We almost always end up moving from kettlebells to dumbbells. Our heaviest kettlebell is 46 kilograms (about 100 pounds). Our heaviest dumbbell is 120 pounds.

FEET-ELEVATED DUMBBELL DEADLIFT
PROGRESSION 2

Once athletes can handle 120 pounds (55 kg) (or your heaviest dumbbell), elevate the feet on six-inch (15 cm) boxes to increase the range of motion. This gives three to four more weeks of progression. Generally when we add range we go down about 20 pounds (10 kg), so 120 × 5 becomes 100 × 5.

TRAP-BAR OR HEX-BAR DEADLIFT

PROGRESSION 3

The trap-bar or hex-bar deadlift (figure 6.13) joins the kettlebell deadlift and goblet squat in our big three bilateral exercises. Where the kettlebell deadlift and goblet squat can be viewed as basic beginner exercises, the trap-bar deadlift can be used as a major bilateral strength exercise.

The trap bar is a great invention that allows a deadlift action (weight in the hands) in combination with more of a squat pattern (deep movement of the knees and hips). In effect the bar passes through the body, so the issue of pulling a straight bar off the floor and having to move around the knees is eliminated. This eliminates the shear forces that can make the deadlift problematic for some lifters.

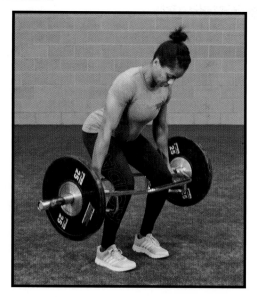

Figure 6.13 Trap-bar or hex-bar deadlift.

The trap bar can also be used in more of a conventional deadlift pattern (deep movement of the hips with limited knee bend) or a modified straight-leg deadlift pattern. The trap bar is a really valuable tool because it allows bilateral total-body exercise that is safer on the back than squatting when done properly.

The key to understanding why the deadlift may be less stressful on the lower back than squats strangely enough relates to shoulder mobility. The compensation for poor shoulder mobility is lumbar extension. Poor shoulder mobility is a major causative factor in back pain. If an athlete tries to place a bar on the shoulders to squat but lacks shoulder mobility, what does he do? He extends the lumbar spine. If he tries to get his elbows up in a front squat and lacks shoulder mobility, what does he do? He extends the lumbar spine.

Just as the hips and spine are linked, so are the lumbar spine and the shoulders. Next time you have an athlete with low back pain, don't just look at hip mobility; look at shoulder mobility and at exercise selection. This is why low back pain is less common in the deadlift versus the squat. The elimination of forced external rotation in those who lack it may cause a significant decrease in back symptoms. It's amazing what you learn when you listen and think.

The trap-bar deadlift is what we called a hybrid exercise in the first edition of *Functional Training for Sports*, a cross between a squat and a deadlift. In any case, it is simple to teach and safer than the conventional deadlift because of the design of the bar. The diamond-shaped trap bar allows the athlete to begin inside and simply stand up with the weight. Unlike in conventional deadlifts, stress can be kept off the back because the athlete can sit more than lean. The trap bar does not require keeping the bar close to the shins and thus eliminates many of the potential hazards of the conventional deadlift.

DELOADING THE SQUAT PATTERN

REGRESSION 3

If goblet squats fail to produce acceptable technique, another option, particularly for older clients, may be to deload the squat pattern. Some older clients or injured athletes may simply be too weak to properly execute the squat pattern. Deloading allows work at less than body weight without resorting to machines such as the leg press. Deloading can be done with any suspension device (e.g., rings, TRX) or any pull-down machine. Load is added by either using less upper body assistance (in the case of rings or TRX) or by decreasing the weight on the pull-down machine. I prefer the pull-down machine because it allows you to quantify the decrease in assistance.

After appropriate movement is mastered at some level, it's time to add load. There are many tools for load, including but not limited to barbells, kettlebells, dumbbells, rocks, and bricks, but remember: Appropriate movement first.

DEVELOPING SINGLE-LEG STRENGTH

The process of developing single-leg strength has advanced significantly in the past decade. Ten years ago it was rare to see an athlete perform a functional single-leg exercise. In fact, many coaches ridiculed single-leg exercises such as lunges and single-leg squat variations. If an athlete performed single-leg exercises, they were often unilateral machine-based exercises such as unilateral leg presses or unilateral leg extensions and leg curls. Now some coaches have completely abandoned conventional double-leg exercises in favor of a program of strictly single-leg versions, especially for athletes with lower back problems or athletes who are skeptical about strength training. Many athletes in sports that traditionally have not emphasized heavy strength training have a closed-minded approach to exercises such as back squats and power cleans but are very open to the idea of single-leg strength and plyometrics. Single-leg training allows aggressive lower body work for athletes who might otherwise avoid strength training entirely.

Although it has been ignored in conventional strength programs, single-leg strength may actually be essential for the improvement of speed and balance and the prevention of injury. Single-leg strength is the essence of functional lower body strength training; a case can be made that all double-leg exercises are nonfunctional for most sports.

Although viewing bilateral squatting and deadlifting as nonfunctional may be considered extreme, the claim illustrates the need for single-leg exercises in any strength program. Unfortunately, many strength programs still focus exclusively on conventional double-leg exercises, such as squats and deadlifts, or worse still on completely nonfunctional leg exercises such as leg presses, leg extensions, and leg curls.

To properly frame the functional versus nonfunctional debate, go back to a simple question we asked early in this book. How many sports are played with both feet in contact with the ground at the same time? The answer is one: Rowers produce force simultaneously with both legs. However, most sports skills are performed on one leg. For this simple reason, it is critical that single-leg strength be a focal point of the strength program.

Single-leg strength is specific and cannot be developed through double-leg exercises. The actions of the pelvic stabilizers are different in a single-leg stance than in a double-leg stance. Single-leg exercises force the gluteus medius (a muscle in the buttocks), adductors, and quadratus lumborum (a lower back muscle) to operate as stabilizers, which are critical in sports skills. These muscles (gluteus medius, adductors, quadratus lumborum) do not need to perform their stabilizer role in conventional double-leg exercises. In addition, single-leg strength is now recognized as a key in injury reduction and has become a staple of all rehabilitation, reconditioning, and knee injury prevention programs.

These single-leg exercises are classified as baseline, as progressions (1, 2, 3, or 4), or as regressions from the baseline. All athletes, regardless of training stage, should begin with the appropriate baseline exercise for the first three weeks of training. Almost all progression 2 exercises can be done with some type of external load by more advanced athletes, but remember that athletes should progress only when they have mastered an exercise. After athletes have mastered a baseline single-leg strength exercise, they can progress to the next single-leg strength exercise in the progression.

Most of the single-leg exercises can initially use a simple body-weight progression. This means the athlete uses body weight only (no external weight) for the first three weeks but increases reps each week from 8 to 10 to 12 per leg. This is a simple progressive resistance concept. More advanced athletes might want to begin with external loads (bar, dumbbells, or weight vest), but this is discouraged initially if the athletes do not have experience with single-leg training. As athletes become more advanced, any single-leg exercise can be added into the program as long as no fewer than five reps are used.

▶ SPLIT SQUAT
BASELINE

The split squat (see figure 6.14) might be the best exercise for developing single-leg strength. Split squats are both easy to perform and easy to learn, so it is always step 1 in our single-leg progression. We have regressions and progressions, but our baseline exercise is the split squat.

To perform the split squat, assume a split-stance position with the feet in line with the shoulders and about three to four feet (1 to 1.2 m) apart. This position provides two solid, stable points on the ground. For body-weight split squats, clasp the hands behind the head or place the hands on your hips. From this position drop the back knee down to the floor (or an Airex pad) while keeping the weight over the heel of the front foot. It is critical to cue the back knee down and weight on the front heel. You do not want a big forward weight shift onto the ball of the foot. The knee can move forward over the toes as long as the weight stays on the heel of the front foot.

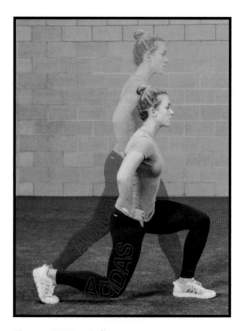

Figure 6.14   Split squat.

Teaching Cue

Tampa-based strength and conditioning coach Brad Kaczmarski gave us a great suggestion to help teach the split squat. Kaczmarski suggests using a "bottom up" approach, and this is one of the first things we do if an athlete struggles to learn the movement. To teach bottom up, simply get the athlete into a kneeling lunge stretch position and have her push up through the back heel. Cueing "bottom up" quickly cures athletes who struggle with the back hip position or core control.

Please note that the split squat is not a lunge. The exercise involves no foot movement or stepping. Split squats have the added benefit of developing balance and dynamic flexibility in the hip flexor muscles.

Technique Points

- Concentrate on dropping the back knee down to the floor with the weight on the front heel.
- Keep the head and chest up. A position with the hands behind the head works best for beginners.
- Think of the back foot as a balance point. Don't attempt to use the back leg.
- Think *bottom up* if athletes struggle.
- The knee of the back leg should be slightly flexed. A *slight* hip flexor stretch will be felt in the bottom when positioned correctly.

Initial loading for all these single-leg exercises is best done in the previously described goblet position. Load in the goblet position until the athlete struggles to get the dumbbell into place (two contact points), and then switch to a side-loading position with two dumbbells.

Note: For a number of years we quickly switched from split squats to rear-foot-elevated split squats. In retrospect this may have been a mistake. The quick switch was made because athletes complained about the pressure on the big toe of the back foot as the loads got heavy. So we switched everyone and then realized we should continue with the split squat until the athlete complains of big toe discomfort instead of simply split-squatting for three weeks and then jumping quickly to a more advanced variation. We have found that our athletes get very strong in the split squat with no complaints.

REAR-FOOT-ELEVATED SPLIT SQUAT
PROGRESSION 1

The rear-foot-elevated split squat has been the primary lower body strength exercise in our program for the last five years. We use conventional split squats for at least the first six weeks before switching to the rear-foot-elevated version.

For the rear-foot-elevated split squat (see figure 6.15), get into a position similar to that for the split squat, except place the back foot on a bench or a specially designed rounded stand. The foot must be placed with the shoelaces down. Do not allow athletes to place the toe on the bench. Athletes will not be able to handle heavy loads in the rear-foot-elevated split squat if they attempt to balance on the toe.

In this position there is still one stable point of support on the floor, but now there is one slightly less stable point on the bench or stand. This is a fairly significant increase in difficulty from the split squat because the back leg now provides less stability and assistance. From this position, descend until the front thigh is parallel to the floor and the back knee is nearly touching the floor. Like the split squat, this exercise is done with no foot movement, and it also improves the dynamic flexibility of the hip flexor muscles.

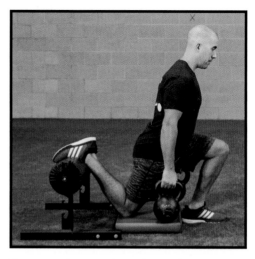

Figure 6.15   Rear-foot-elevated split squat.

This exercise can begin as a body-weight exercise, following the 8-10-12 body-weight progression described earlier, but it is best used as a strength exercise with dumbbells or kettlebells. Begin loading with a dumbbell in the goblet position. Continue to goblet load as long as the athlete can move the dumbbell into place (two contact points). Our male athletes have used in excess of 100 pounds (45 kg), and our females routinely use 50 to 60 pounds (23 to 27 kg) before switching loading styles. Kettlebells work extremely well from a grip and balance standpoint once athletes can no longer goblet load. We will go as low as five reps per leg per set (e.g., three sets of five reps per leg). Athletes will quickly get to the point where they are using the heaviest dumbbells or kettlebells available. Weight vests can add additional load as needed. Loads in the rear-foot-elevated split squat will need to be 30 to 40 pounds (13 to 18 kg) less than loads in the preceding split squat. This means the progression in exercise difficulty results in a regression in load.

To provide a perspective on loading, we have female athletes who can perform 10 reps with 36-kilogram kettlebells (80 pounds per hand) and male athletes who can use 120-pound (55 kg) dumbbells in each hand for 10 reps.

SINGLE-LEG SQUAT
PROGRESSION 2

The single-leg squat (see figure 6.16) is the king of single-leg exercises. It may be the most difficult but is also probably the most beneficial. The single-leg squat requires the use of a single leg without any contribution to balance or stability from the opposite leg. Unlike the kickstand-like effect of the back foot in the split-squat variations, the pelvic muscles must function as stabilizers without the benefit of the opposite leg touching the ground or a bench. The importance of this point cannot be overstated, as pelvic or hip stability is needed in all sprinting actions. In sprinting, the stance leg must produce force without any assistance from the swing leg.

Some athletes are unable to perform this exercise immediately and should not become discouraged. Most athletes feel unsteady or clumsy the first few times, and it might take a few sessions to become comfortable. One of the major benefits of single-leg squats is the sense of balance they develop.

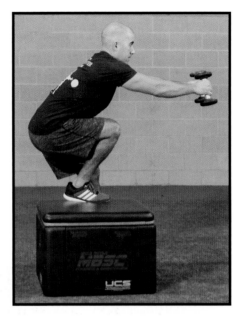

Figure 6.16   Single-leg squat on a plyo box.

Note: Single-leg squats should *not* be confused with pistol squats. We neither do nor endorse pistol squats for a number of reasons. Although these two exercises seem very similar, they are not interchangeable. In the single-leg squat there is significantly less stress on the hip flexors and subsequently less stress on the lower back than in a pistol squat. Working off a box versus off the floor allows the free leg to drop lower. Pistol squats can often cause low back pain due to overuse of the hip flexors to hold the free leg extended and parallel to the floor. In addition, the single-leg squat is done to a thigh-parallel position. No attempt is made to go below parallel. Below-parallel squatting often results in lumbar rounding and may cause the posterior aspects of the medial meniscus to be compressed in the joint line. Remember, during flexion of the knee the meniscus moves forward in the joint, and the posterior aspect of the meniscus (the posterior horn) can be pinched in below-parallel squatting.

Technique Points

- Stand on a plyometric box or bench holding a pair of 5-pound (2.5 kg) dumbbells. This is the second case in which a load makes the lift easier. The counterbalance of 5 pounds in each hand makes performing a single-leg squat easier than if it were done without weight. Attempt to lower to a position with the thigh parallel to the floor. Although the dumbbells may not seem like a good idea, the counterbalance definitely makes the movement easier to learn.

- While beginning to lower into the squat, raise the dumbbells to shoulder level to facilitate sitting back on the heel.

- Concentrate on keeping the weight on the heel to minimize movement at the ankle and to keep the knee from moving beyond the big toe in the bottom position. Standing with the heel on a plate or specially made wedge can be extremely helpful.

- It is critical to begin by bending at the knee and not by bending at the ankle. Watch carefully for this.

Most athletes should begin with three sets of five reps with 5-pound dumbbells. Progress by increasing reps or by increasing the weight of the dumbbells, depending on the stage of the training cycle (e.g., strength phase or accumulation phase). As with the rear-foot-elevated split squat, do no fewer than five reps per leg.

PARTIAL SINGLE-LEG SQUAT
REGRESSION 1

The single-leg squat is one of the few exercises that can be done for less than the described range of motion. Although partial-range exercises are generally avoided, the value in the exercise from a hip and pelvic stability standpoint is so great that it is well worth teaching clients or athletes who are unable to perform the exercise as deeply as possible (until parallel is reached). I call this progressive range of motion training. Instead of progressive resistance, the resistance (body weight plus 5 pounds in each hand) is kept constant while the athlete or client works to attain the desired range. We generally stack Airex pads to increase or decrease depth.

SINGLE-LEG DEADLIFT
REGRESSION 2

In the first edition of *Functional Training for Sports* we called this exercise a skater's single-leg squat. We used this term because the exercise was described as a hockey-specific version of the single-leg box squat. Instead of keeping the torso erect and placing the free leg out in front, the torso is brought down to touch the thigh (see figure 6.17) and the

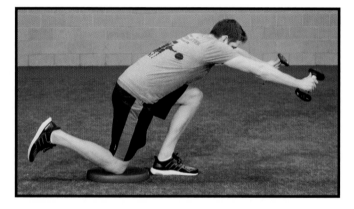

Figure 6.17   Single-leg deadlift.

free leg is bent at the knee. This forward flexed position simulates a skater's starting position. However, as our thought process on squats and deadlifts changed, we realized this exercise has deep hip movement and should be classified as a deadlift. In fact, if observed from the side the joint angles are nearly identical to the trap-bar deadlift.

The single-leg deadlift is an excellent alternative for those who cannot deadlift because of low back issues. It is not the single-leg straight-leg deadlift presented later, although the exercises have shared movement of the hip and knee. This is the third exercise that actually seems better with load. Begin with 5-pound (2.5 kg) dumbbells in the hands, as in the single-leg squat.

Follow the 8-10-12 body-weight progression, and then add weight with a combination of dumbbells and weight vests.

LUNGE
PROGRESSION 3

The lunge (see figure 6.18) is another great single-leg exercise. It is mistakenly considered by many to be an easy alternative to the squat. In fact, the lunge is a big soreness producer and does not fall in the easy category at all. The key benefit of the lunge, and the reason it is an advanced exercise, is that the lower body muscles must work to decelerate the body as it moves forward. The lunge is an advanced progression because the body must be properly prepared for the deceleration component. In addition, lunges are an excellent dynamic stretching movement for the hip area and can be included in both strength training and warm-up routines for this reason alone. Athletes who have had groin or hip flexor problems will find the lunge a very beneficial exercise.

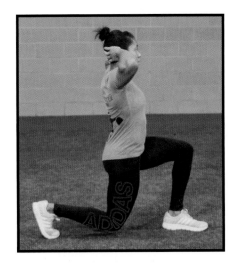

Figure 6.18   Lunge.

Technique Points

- The back should stay tight and slightly arched, and the upper body should stay erect.
- The movement begins in standing with the feet together.
- The step should be just slightly shorter than the athlete is tall. The step should be long enough to slightly stretch the hip flexor muscles of the rear leg.
- The movement is a step forward one with a "push back" action and ends with the feet back together.

As many as 10 reps on each leg can be done for endurance. Lunges can be included in leg circuits in combination with other exercises.

SLIDE-BOARD LUNGE
PROGRESSION 3A

The slide-board lunge is an excellent single-leg exercise that combines single-leg strength, dynamic flexibility, and moderate instability. This is a great movement for both training and rehabilitation. To keep from monopolizing the slide boards, this exercise can be done on a four-foot (1.2 m) length of slide-board-top material rather than a slide board itself or, with a Valslide. Wear one slide-board shoe on the back foot, and slide the foot back in a back lunge (see figure 6.19). The back foot slides forward and back while the

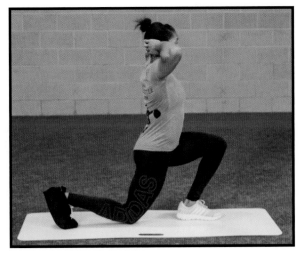

Figure 6.19   Slide-board lunge.

front foot performs a single-leg squat. Place the hands behind the head, and keep the front knee over the midfoot.

This is a very interesting exercise. It looks like a split squat, but the pulling action probably places it in the posterior-chain category with exercises such as the single-leg straight-leg deadlift. A hip-dominant exercise that looks like a knee-dominant exercise is a great choice if you can do only one lower body movement. One drawback of the slide-board lunge is that we have not had great experiences with heavy loads. The effectiveness of the exercise seems to be compromised when used as a strength exercise, so it is best done in early phases of hypertrophy and anatomical adaption.

Use a body-weight progression with this exercise because of the additional stretch and instability component.

LATERAL SQUAT
PROGRESSION 3B

The lateral body-weight squat can be used both as a warm-up exercise and as a strength exercise. It is an excellent exercise to promote dynamic flexibility of the adductor musculature and to improve strength for athletes who move in the frontal plane such as baseball players or hockey players. Stand with the feet approximately four feet (1.2 m) apart and sit to one side (see figure 6.20). Keep the weight on the heel as you sit, and keep the knee over the toe. Wider is better in this exercise. Athletes taller than five feet eight inches (173 cm) will have difficulty performing this exercise with their feet less than four feet apart.

Use the body-weight progression for the lateral squat.

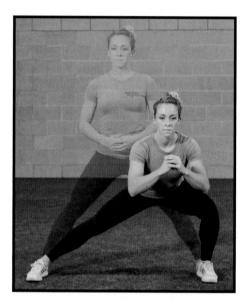

Figure 6.20   Lateral squat.

LATERAL LUNGE
PROGRESSION 4

The lateral lunge is a decelerative exercise done in the frontal plane. In other words, the body moves side to side. Athletes who have learned the lateral squat will progress seamlessly to the lateral lunge. Both lateral lunges and lateral squats can be used as either dynamic warm-ups or as strength exercises.

THUMBS DOWN ON STEP-UPS

The step-up can be an alternative to the squat, but step-ups may cause more discomfort for athletes with knee problems than any of the previously mentioned single-leg exercises because of the lack of an initial eccentric contraction. The step-up is not a preferred single-leg movement because athletes can cheat too easily by pushing off with the foot on the ground.

IMPROVING SINGLE-LEG STABILITY

Athletes often perform exercises such as the split squat and single-leg bench squat reasonably well but struggle with true single-leg squats. Frequently these are the same athletes who suffer from knee problems such as chondromalacia patellae (softening of the knee cartilage), patellar tendinitis, or other patellofemoral syndromes. In my experience, these athletes generally share a common difficulty in stabilizing the lower extremity while squatting because of a weak lateral hip. The gluteus medius is an often-neglected muscle of the hip whose primary function is to stabilize the lower extremity in single-leg movements such as running, jumping, and squatting.

In many athletes this muscle is either too weak to perform its function or is not "turned on" neurologically. As a result, the support structures of the knee are forced to provide stability instead of the gluteus medius. This may mean pain in the iliotibial band, in the patellar tendon, or under the kneecap. For many years these problems were blamed on poor quadriceps strength, and doctors and therapists prescribed simple nonfunctional exercise such as leg extensions to solve the problem. Recently therapists and athletic trainers have begun to recognize the role of the lateral glutes in these knee problems.

We have found two ways to turn on these muscles: mini-band side steps and cross-body reaching.

MINI-BAND WALKS

Mini-band walks are an easy way to turn on the lateral glutes. The athlete simply places the band around the ankles and moves laterally. With mini-band walks both hips are abducting simultaneously, the stance leg is a closed chain (foot in contact with the ground), and the other is in open-chain abduction. There are two big keys to mini-band work:

- Maintain band tension. The feet must be kept far enough apart to keep the band tight.
- Don't rock. Often people with weak lateral glutes will rock side to side instead of stepping laterally.

To stimulate the hip rotator group, place the band on the feet. Placing the band on the feet instead of at the ankles creates an internal rotation force and results in greater stimulation of the hip external rotators.

CROSS-BODY REACHING

Cross-body reaching can be used in any knee- or hip-dominant exercise to facilitate more glute involvement. Reaching across the working leg increases the contribution of the glutes. The complicated anatomical explanation is that the pelvis rotates against the fixed femur, resulting in internal rotation of the hip. Because the glutes are external rotators, they are stretched and respond with a greater contribution. This will result in more hip stability. Interestingly enough, many see hip stability as knee stability and describe instability as the "the knee caving in." In reality the knee valgus is hip adduction and internal rotation and is really not a knee issue at all.

HIP EXTENSIONS AND HEALTHY HAMSTRINGS

As mentioned previously, the muscles that extend the hip, primarily the gluteus maximus and hamstring group, are still neglected in many training programs. Many programs place excessive emphasis on the squat and squat variations and neglect the hip extensors.

In programming it is important to understand that knee-dominant exercises such as squats and the single-leg squat variations affect the glutes and hamstrings differently than the hip-dominant exercises that John and Tsatsouline describe in *Easy Strength* as having deep hip movement with minimal knee bend. Although our functional anatomy concept tells us all muscles are involved in every lower body exercise, the degree to which the hips and knees bend can determine areas of emphasis or concentration. To more fully involve the glutes and the hamstrings, the movement must be centered on the hip and not on the knee.

To understand this concept, envision a single-leg squat. The hip moves through an approximately 90-degree range of motion in concert with the knee. Generally there is 1 degree of hip movement for each degree of knee movement. The focus of the exercise is shared equally by the knee extensors and the hip extensors, and there is deep movement of the knees *and* hips. In an exercise such as the single-leg straight-leg deadlift, the hip moves through a 90-degree range of motion while the knee maintains a slight 10- to 20-degree knee bend. This is deep movement of the hips. A properly designed program must include a balance of knee-dominant exercises and hip-dominant exercises.

Single-Leg Hip-Dominant Progressions

There may be nothing more important than unilateral hip dominant exercises for improving performance and preventing hamstring injury. I might go so far as to say that exercises like one leg straight leg deadlifts and it's variations are the most important exercises in the lower body program. The major reason for this might be that the posterior chain is so often neglected in conventional strength programs. You rarely hear about a pulled quadriceps in sports but, pulled hamstrings are very common. Don't overlook this critical area when designing a functional strength program.

SINGLE-LEG STRAIGHT-LEG DEADLIFT
BASELINE

The single-leg straight-leg deadlift has become the king of posterior-chain exercises. It not only develops the entire posterior chain (glutes, hamstrings, and long adductors) but also enhances balance. This exercise is safe, challenging, and extremely beneficial and is the classic illustration of what we referred to previously as deep hip movement with minimal knee movement. The currently fashionable term that best describes the motion of the single-leg straight-leg deadlift is the concept of hip hinge. Hip hinging is the ability to move from the hip without flexing the lumbar spine. The knees are bent 10 to 20 degrees, with all remaining motion coming from the hip. The key is zero flexion of the lumbar spine. This motion is frequently referred to as a "golfer's lift" because the action resembles the motion used to retrieve a tee from the grass.

If I can program only two lower body exercises, they will almost always be split squats and single-leg straight-leg deadlifts. If I am starting a beginner on a program, I will start with the same two. The single-leg straight-leg deadlift is preferred in our programs over any double-leg posterior-chain versions. Single-leg posterior-chain work is obviously more functional than double-leg posterior-chain work, and single-leg posterior-chain work that also challenges balance and proprioception is the most beneficial. One of the secondary benefits of the single-leg straight-leg deadlift is the tremendous proprioceptive work at the ankle. Other pluses are that high loads are not necessary and the possibility of back injury is almost nonexistent.

This is another exercise, like the lateral squat, that can and will be used as both a body-weight warm-up and as a loaded strength exercise. On the days we don't do split squats and single-leg straight-leg deadlifts with loads for strength, we do them as body-weight exercises for mobility work and warm-up.

It is important to note that this is designed to eventually become a strength exercise. We have had athletes use upwards of 225 pounds (100 kg) in the single-leg straight-leg deadlift.

Technique Points

- A single kettlebell or dumbbell is held in the hand opposite the foot on the floor. (Kettlebells are preferred because they are easy to hold and create a consistent downward force.) Lean forward from the hip while lifting the free leg to the rear in line with the torso. Think about moving as one long piece from head to toe (see figure 6.21). Keep the chest up and the lower back flat.

- *Attempt* to place the kettlebell or dumbbell on the ground just inside the grounded foot.

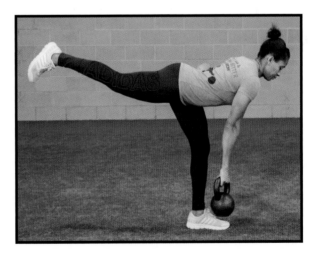

Figure 6.21   Single-leg straight-leg deadlift.

- Think about getting as long as possible through the back leg. Think back toes up to the shin and back heel pressing into an imaginary wall behind.
- The goal of the exercise is not to get the kettlebell or dumbbell to the floor. Focus on the sensation of a hamstring stretch to reinforce proper technique.
- Big tip: If the knee caves in, try to reach across to the outside of the foot. This rotational action rotates the pelvis against the femur and stretches the glute.

Do two or three sets of 5 to 10 reps per leg, depending on training level and phase of training.

REACHING SINGLE-LEG STRAIGHT-LEG DEADLIFT
REGRESSION 1

The reaching version of the single-leg straight-leg deadlift (see figure 6.22) is an excellent way to regress those who struggle to learn what is now commonly referred to as the hip hinge. Many beginner trainees will struggle to move from the hip and will want to move from the lumbar spine. Many will also initially struggle with balance.

The reaching version begins with no weight and is best done to a cone, which will encourage and reinforce the reaching action. The key in the reaching version is again to get as long as possible, but this time the instruction is to reach back with the free foot

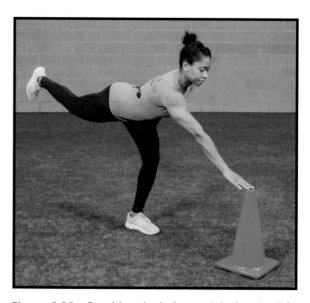

Figure 6.22   Reaching single-leg straight-leg deadlift.

while reaching forward with the hand. This exercise is close to foolproof because the extension of the back leg turns on the glutes and hamstrings of the free leg, while the reaching of the hand turns on both the lumbar and thoracic extensors. Athletes and clients can progress to a light handled medicine balls in the hand, but the initial teaching requires only body weight. This exercise can become the baseline exercise for younger (11 or 12) or older (30-plus) clients.

Technique Points

- Think toes up to shins and hands reaching as far forward as possible.
- Get as long as possible. Long is the big cue, and cueing "long" will prevent lumbar flexion and encourage hip hinging.
- Loading can be done via a medicine ball in the hand. Light handled medicine balls work particularly well.

CROSS-REACHING SINGLE-LEG STRAIGHT-LEG DEADLIFT
REGRESSION 2

If the reaching regression does not work, it is often because the athlete or client cannot properly use the glutes to stabilize the hips. This can lead to several instability and technique errors. To combat this, encourage the athlete or client to again move the pelvis on the fixed femur, described as cross-body reaching in the section on single-leg stability (see figure 6.23). (Don't try to explain the pelvis moving against the femur; just tell the athlete to reach across the body.) The cross-reach drives the pelvis and creates an internal rotation of the pelvis on the fixed femur of the stance leg. The result is a stretch to the glutes, increased recruitment, and increased stability on the stance leg.

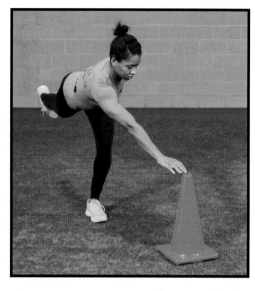

Figure 6.23 Cross-reaching single-leg straight-leg deadlift.

To create this motion, line the athlete up in front of a cone with the cone placed 12"outside the foot on the ground ask her to reach across the body to the opposite-side upright. This is a magic corrective exercise that can often take an unstable, wobbly athlete and create immediate stability. To load use a handled medicine ball.

CABLE LOADED SINGLE-LEG STRAIGHT-LEG DEADLIFT
PROGRESSION 1

The low pulley version of the single-leg straight leg deadlift (see figure 6.24) can be used as a baseline exercise if plenty of low pulley cables are available. In one-to-one situations this might be the best way to initially teach and perform the single-leg straight-leg deadlift pattern. However, for larger groups or teams, this may not be the best practical choice. This exercise can be a load progression and a great teaching tool at the same time because the exercise seems to have a self-correcting component to it.

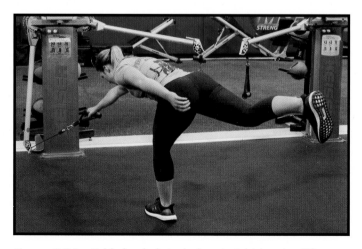

Figure 6.24 Cable loaded single-leg straight-leg deadlift.

The key is the vector of the load resistance. Rather than lowering the load down toward the ground, the trainee is actually pulled forward by the load. This changes the loading of the posterior chain and creates a great pulling, hip extension vector.

- Set up in front of a low pulley with a single handle.
- Gripping hand is opposite of stance foot.
- Again cue "long body" and a very strong hip extension action.
- Front leg continues to be in the 10- to 20-degree knee bend.

BAND LOADED SINGLE-LEG STRAIGHT-LEG DEADLIFT
PROGRESSION 2

This is the same as the previous exercise except the load is provided by a band instead of a low pulley. The advantages here are twofold.

- Exercise bands such as Perform Better Superbands are much less expensive than a low pulley system.
- The resistance increases as the hip moves into extension.

One of the benefits (and potential drawbacks) of band work is that resistance is increased at end range as the band is stretched. This is viewed positively in loading the posterior chain because the greatest stresses on the muscles are at end range as the push-off phase of running begins.

- Execution of the exercise doesn't change. The emphasis is still on getting a long body and hinging from the hip.
- The difference is that the exercise is easiest in the stretched position, and the load increases as the length of the band increases, resulting in maximal loading at hip extension.

LOWER BODY STRENGTH AND POWER
CASE STUDY: GOSDER CHERILUS

The tackle position in football is played by men with basketball height, football size (usually over 300 pounds), and remarkable athleticism. Tampa Bay Buccaneer offensive tackle Gosder Cherilus fits the mold at about six-foot-five (196 cm) and 315 pounds (143 kg). Often the height of these athletes makes exercises such as the squat and deadlift difficult. Taller athletes often struggle with technique in bilateral lifts and can frequently experience back pain. However, exercises such as single-leg squats, split squats, and single-leg straight-leg deadlifts allow these giants to train hard and stay healthy. Gosder has used these functional exercises to keep himself healthy in the NFL for the last five years. Unilateral work can be great for any athlete but is of particular value to larger athletes looking to work around injuries as they age.

The great thing about large men and unilateral training is that their body weight is automatically part of the load. A single-leg squat or split squat done with 10 pounds (5 kg) creates a load of 325 pounds (147 kg). The result is that larger players get an additional benefit from functional training based on their large body weight. An exercise such as a single-leg squat can be a major challenge for a larger athlete who demonstrates great strength with the barbell but lacks relative functional strength.

Bridging Progressions: Learning to Leg Curl

Hip-dominant exercises can be broken down further into those that target the glutes and those that target the hamstrings. Bridges and single-leg bridges are core exercises that can be used initially to target the glutes and then progressed into leg curl variations that target the hamstrings.

To make matters more difficult, the muscles that help extend the hip, especially the hamstrings, are still often mistakenly trained as knee flexors. In many outdated strength programs, some muscle groups are still trained according to antiquated understandings of their function originating from what we described previously as origin–insertion anatomy.

Although some anatomy texts still describe the hamstring group as knee flexors, the hamstrings are actually powerful extensors of the hip and stabilizers of the knee. The hamstrings serve as knee flexors only in nonfunctional settings. In running, jumping, and skating, the function of the hamstrings is not to flex the knee but to extend the hip.

As a result, exercises such as lying or standing leg curls are a waste of time. Machine leg curls exercise the hamstring muscles in a pattern and manner that is never used in sport or in life. The fact that we often train or rehabilitate the hamstring muscles in these nonfunctional patterns may explain the frequent recurrence of hamstring strains in athletes who rehabilitate with exercises such as leg curls.

Please note: Stability ball leg curls and slide-board leg curls, which are illustrated later in this chapter, are an exception because these particular exercises use a closed-chain movement (foot in contact with a supporting surface) and are done in concert with the glutes when performed correctly.

Training the glutes and hamstrings as hip extensors rather than knee flexors goes a long way toward eliminating the hamstring strains so often seen in sport. Athletes and coaches are reminded to think about the true function of the muscles, not the anatomy-book description. Forget about hamstrings as knee flexors. See the hamstrings as powerful hip extensors and as muscles that eccentrically decelerate knee extension in running. Also remember to work the hamstrings and glutes with the knee flexed and the knee extended. This might be a major shift in thinking for some, but it will pay off in healthier hamstrings.

There are a number of names for bridges and bridge progressions. Bridges are also called hip lifts and hip thrusts. I dislike the name *hip thrust* and prefer the term *hip lift*. To me, *thrust* denotes a powerful action that lacks the control so necessary in this exercise. Bridging is the point of crossover from core training to lower body training. The initial stages of bridging are often done in the mobility and activation portion of the program as the athlete or client undertakes the difficult motor learning task of separating hip extension and glute function from lumbar extension. However, the same action progresses into single bridges or single-leg hip lifts and into shoulder-elevated bridges and hip lifts. Eventually the act of bridging forms the beginning of the slide-board or stability ball leg curl.

SINGLE-LEG BRIDGE OR COOK HIP LIFT

BASELINE

Noted physical therapist Gray Cook popularized this exercise to teach athletes how to quickly and easily separate the function of the hip extensors from the lumbar extensors. Most athletes are unaware of how little range of motion they possess in the hip joint when the range of motion in the lumbar spine is intentionally limited. The great thing about properly performed hip lifts or bridges is that you have a core exercise, an active

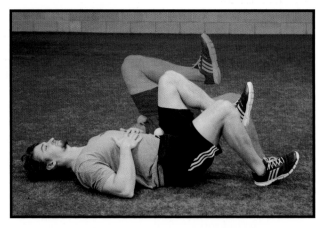

Figure 6.25   Single-leg bridge or Cook hip lift.

stretching exercise, and a glute strength exercise all rolled into one simple movement.

To perform the movement, lie on the back with the feet flat on the floor (hook-lying position). Then place a tennis ball on the low end of the rib cage and pull the knee to the chest hard enough to hold the tennis ball in place. From this position, push down through the foot on the floor and extend the hip while keeping the tennis ball tight against the ribs with the opposite leg (see figure 6.25). The range of motion in this exercise is only two to three inches (5 to 8 cm). The range of motion can be increased significantly by relaxing the grip on the opposite knee, but this defeats the purpose. Relaxing the hold on the leg substitutes lumbar spine extension for hip extension.

This exercise has three distinct benefits.

1. The exercise uses the glutes as the primary hip extensor while decreasing the contribution of the hamstrings as hip extensors.
2. The exercise teaches the athlete how to distinguish between hip extension and lumbar spine extension.
3. The coach or trainer can evaluate tightness in the hip flexor group that may be limiting hip extension and contributing to lower back pain.

If an athlete experiences cramping in the hamstrings, the glutes are not working properly. Physical therapist Mike Clark of the National Academy of Sports Medicine (NASM) uses this as an example of synergistic dominance, in which the hamstrings are forced to compensate for a weak gluteus maximus.

SHOULDER-ELEVATED HIP LIFT

PROGRESSION 1

The shoulder-elevated hip lift is an excellent progression from the Cook hip lift. The shoulders are elevated on a standard exercise bench to increase the difficulty of the exercise.

For all these hip-lift exercises, use the 8-10-12 body-weight progression.

STABILITY BALL LEG CURL ▶

PROGRESSION 2

The stability ball leg curl is an advanced exercise because it requires using the glutes and spinal erectors to stabilize the torso and the hamstrings to perform a closed-chain leg curl. This exercise develops torso stability while also strengthening the hamstrings. The stability ball leg curl and the slide-board leg curl are the only leg curl movements I recommend.

Technique Points

- Heels are placed on the ball, and the body is held with the hips off the ground.
- The ball is curled under the body with the heels while the body is kept straight (see figure 6.26).

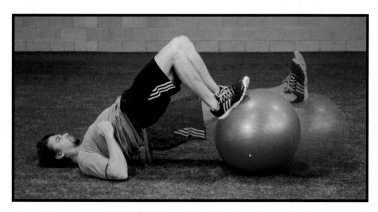

Figure 6.26   Stability ball leg curl.

SLIDE-BOARD LEG CURL

PROGRESSION 3

The slide-board leg curl is identical to the stability ball version except a slide board, mini slide board, or Valslides are used. The action is identical. Slide-board leg curls are more difficult than stability ball leg curls as the stability ball creates a downhill slope.

This chapter describes the foundation of a proper lower body strength program. Learning to squat and performing single-leg exercises are two keys for developing speed and power. Follow the progressions and guidelines given. Don't look for an easy way out by reverting to machine training for the lower body. An athlete cannot develop balance, flexibility, and strength while sitting or lying down. The difficult road is often the best road.

REFERENCES

John, D., and P. Tsatsouline. 2011. *Easy Strength*. St. Paul, MN: Dragon Door.

Klein, K., and F. Allman. 1971. *The Knee in Sports*. Austin, TX: Jenkins.

Kuruganti, U., T. Murphy, and T. Pardy. 2011. Bilateral deficit phenomenon and the role of antagonist muscle activity during maximal isometric knee extensions in young, athletic men. *European Journal of Applied Physiology*. 111 (7): 1533-1539. doi: 10.1007/s00421-010-1752-8.

Core Training

One of the stated purposes of this book is to give you ideas you can immediately put to use. The information in this chapter can be used to improve the health and the core function of any athlete and will be of particular interest to coaches and athletes involved in striking sports such as baseball, golf, tennis, field and ice hockey, and cricket.

The core exercises presented are designed to develop a more stable platform from which to strike or throw an object. In addition, the core programs will help any athlete who suffers from low back pain. The medicine ball exercises will improve the power and coordination of all the muscle groups used in striking and throwing skills. Core training is the missing link to developing the power to hit a baseball or golf ball farther or a hockey puck or tennis ball harder and faster. In addition, core training may be a key to a long and healthy sports career.

Any training that works the abdominals, hips, and even scapulothoracic stabilizers can be viewed as core training. In fact, the best functional core exercises may be many of the unilateral knee- and hip-dominant exercises discussed in other sections of this book.

The word *core* is broad by intention to include all muscles in the body's midsection. The core muscles include the

- rectus abdominis (abdominal muscle);
- transversus abdominis (abdominal muscle);
- multifidus muscles (back muscles);
- internal and external obliques (abdominal muscles);
- quadratus lumborum (a low back muscle);
- spinal erectors (back muscles); and to some extent the
- gluteal, hamstring, and hip rotator groups (which cross the hip joint).

These muscles are the vital link between upper body strength and lower body strength. And yet, despite this critical role, core muscles are often trained in an unintelligent, scientifically unsound manner with no real regard for the actual functions of the muscles involved. Furthermore, many commonly used and prescribed core exercises may exacerbate back pain rather than prevent or relieve it.

In the past core training consisted primarily of flexion–extension exercises for the rectus abdominis muscles such as crunches or sit-ups, and the need for a stable and powerful link from the lower body to the upper body was never addressed. Core training is done poorly primarily because it has always been done that way. This leads us back to Lee Cockrell's idea from *Creating Magic*: "What if the way we have always done it is wrong?"

CORE FUNCTION

To truly understand core training, think back to the information on functional anatomy in chapter 1. The abdominal muscles by design are stabilizers, not movers. Even if these muscles were movers, ask yourself how many sports or sporting activities involve flexion and extension of the trunk. The answer, if you really know sport, is very few. Sport is about core stabilization and hip rotation. Are the core muscles actually flexors or rotators of the trunk?

Functional anatomy has demonstrated that the primary purpose of the core musculature is the prevention of motion. In fact, noted physical therapist Shirley Sahrmann in her landmark work *Diagnosis and Treatment of Movement Impairment Syndromes* says, "During most activities, the primary role of the abdominal muscles is to provide isometric support and *limit* the degree of rotation of the trunk" (2002, 70). In much the same way, noted low back researchers James Porterfield and Carl DeRosa state, "Rather than considering the abdominals as flexors and rotators of the trunk—for which they certainly have the capacity—their function might be better viewed as *antirotators and antilateral* flexors of the trunk" (1998, 99). These two relatively simple thoughts totally changed my view on core training as I began to see the core muscles for what they really were rather than what I had been told they were in my 1980 anatomy class. Instead of seeing the muscles as trunk flexors and lateral flexors and prescribing exercises such as crunches and side bends, I now see them as antiextensors and antilateral flexors and more importantly can now envision a concept that has come to be called antirotation. Core training is really about motion prevention, not motion creation.

Over the past two decades strength and conditioning training has moved from a sagittal-plane orientation to an emphasis on unilateral training and multiplanar training. Part of this process, particularly for athletes, has been a misdirected push toward developing spinal mobility in rotation. Any athlete competing in a sport requiring rotation, such as baseball, hockey, and golf, was often blindly urged to develop more range of motion in rotation.

Like many other strength and conditioning coaches, I initially fell victim to this same flawed premise. I was one of the lemmings I dislike so much, blindly following the recommendations of others and using exercises I would now consider questionable or dangerous. Even as a back pain sufferer, I simply wrote off my discomfort as age related and continued to perform rotary stretches and rotary dynamic warm-up exercises.

The aforementioned Shirley Sahrmann (as well as others such as Stuart McGill and Phillip Beach) made me reconsider my position and eventually eliminate a whole group of stretches and dynamic warm-up exercises that were once staples of our programs. As Sahrmann stated in her book, "A large percentage of low back problems occur because the abdominal muscles are not maintaining tight control over the rotation between the pelvis and the spine at the L5-S1 level" (71). The lumbar range of motion that many personal trainers and coaches have attempted to create may not even be desirable and is in fact potentially injurious.

The ability to resist or prevent rotation may be more important than the ability to create it. Clients or athletes must be able to prevent rotation before we should allow them to produce it.

Sahrmann goes on to note a key fact I believe has been overlooked in the performance field. "The overall range of lumbar rotation is . . . approximately 13 degrees. The rotation between each segment from T10 to L5 is 2 degrees. The greatest rotational range is between L5 and S1, which is 5 degrees. . . . The thoracic spine, not the lumbar spine should be the site of greatest amount of rotation of the trunk." When a person practices rotational exercises, he should be instructed to "think about the motion occurring in the area of the chest" (61-62).

Sahrmann places the final icing on the cake with these statements: "Rotation of the lumbar spine is more dangerous than beneficial and rotation of the pelvis and lower extremities to one side while the trunk remains stable or is rotated to the other side is particularly dangerous" (72; see figures 7.1 and 7.2).

Interestingly enough, Sahrmann agrees with the conclusions of noted sprint coach Barry Ross. Ross recommends primarily isometric abdominal training for his sprinters. Sahrmann concurs: "During most activities, the primary role of the abdominal muscles is to provide isometric support and limit the degree of rotation of the trunk which, as discussed, is limited in the lumbar spine" (70).

What does all this mean? It means we need to eliminate stretches and exercises that attempt to increase lumbar range of motion. This includes seated trunk rotational stretches (figure 7.1) and lying trunk rotational stretches.

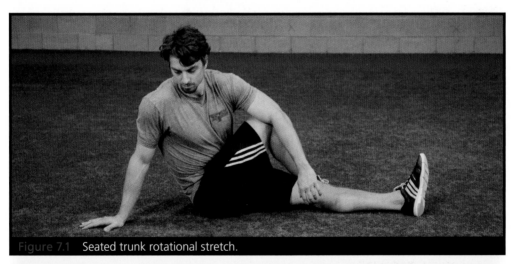

Figure 7.1   Seated trunk rotational stretch.

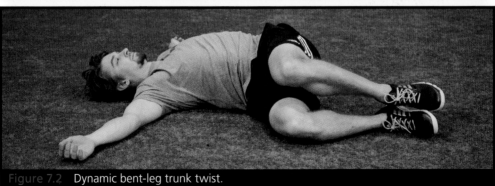

Figure 7.2   Dynamic bent-leg trunk twist.

We must also eliminate dynamic exercises designed to increase trunk range of motion, such as the dynamic bent-leg trunk twist (figure 7.2), the dynamic straight-leg trunk twist (figure 7.3), and the scorpion (figure 7.4).

Most people don't need additional trunk range of motion in the lumbar spine. What we really need is to be able to control the range we have. We have seen a significant decrease in the complaints of low back pain since eliminating the exercises just illustrated. We now emphasize developing hip range of motion in both internal and external rotation.

In the future we will see coaches working on core stability and hip mobility instead of working against themselves by simultaneously trying to develop core range of motion and core stability.

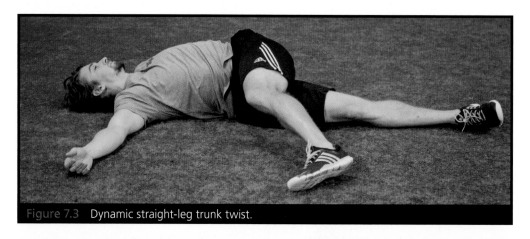

Figure 7.3   Dynamic straight-leg trunk twist.

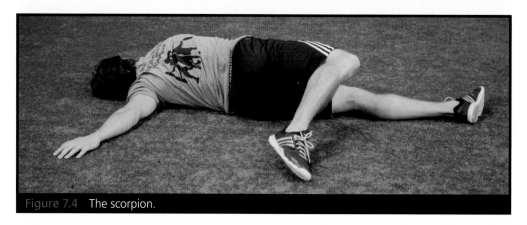

Figure 7.4   The scorpion.

CORE TRAINING IN THE PROGRAM

The subject of when to do core work in the program is frequently debated. Those in favor of core work at the end of the training program cite the possibility of fatiguing the muscles important for stability before the workout. Some are in favor of doing core work before training at least partially to show its importance. The thought is that placing core work at the beginning of the workout establishes the core as a key area for sport training, sort of a first-things-first approach. In past years, that was the approach we favored. Our current approach is to place core exercises throughout the workout, almost as an active rest component.

The main thing is that core work be made a priority and placed intelligently into the workout where appropriate. Another important point to realize is that core work is not like maximal strength work. Many core exercises are isometric in nature and will probably do more to activate or upregulate muscles than to fatigue them. I like to think of exercises that activate or upregulate muscles like using a dimmer switch for a light. You are simply turning up the power to muscles that should be (and are) already working.

Core training may not work the "mirror" muscles as bench presses or curls do, but it is one of the keys to injury reduction and improved sport performance. Remember that a strong core has nothing to do with low body fat. Abdominal definition is the result of diet, not core work. Athletes might train the core muscles to help them shoot harder, throw farther, or stay healthy longer, but for the muscles they've developed to be visible, they need to watch what they eat.

Core Exercise Categories

There are three basic classes of core exercises.

1. *Antiextension* is the primary function of the anterior core muscles and should be addressed in the first two or three phases of all programs. For decades we have developed the anterior core via flexion (bringing the shoulders toward the hips as in a crunch or sit-up, or the hips to the shoulders as in a knee-up or reverse crunch). We now realize that these muscles are stabilizers designed to maintain a stable pelvis under a stable rib cage and must be trained as stabilizers, not as trunk flexors.

2. *Antilateral flexion* develops the quadratus lumborum as well as the obliques as stabilizers of the pelvis and hips, not as lateral flexors of the trunk. Similar to the antiextension concept, varying isometric challenges are employed to work the lateral stabilizers.

3. *Antirotation* might be the key to core training. Antirotation strength is developed through progressions of antiextension exercises and through the use of diagonal patterns and rotational forces. The program contains no rotational exercises, such as trunk twists, Russian twists, or twisting sit-ups.

Breathing and Core Training

The first edition of *Functional Training for Sports* leaned heavily on two sources when it came to guidelines for training the core: Paul Hodges and the Australian physical therapists, who initially gave us many of our stabilization concepts, and Mike Clark of NASM, who popularized the concept of drawing in. Since then there has been a long-running "who's right?" debate about core work, core stabilization, and the concepts of bracing and drawing in. Rather than getting tied up in that debate, I adopted a "whatever works, just get tight" approach and let the experts in academia compete to prove their particular theories right.

Then, in 2014, I was fortunate to meet a physical therapy assistant named Michael Mullin who was trained by a group from Lincoln, Nebraska, called the Postural Restoration Institute. Mullin's teaching offered a simple explanation of breathing, the process of respiration, and how it relates to the concepts of core training and core stability. This fundamentally changed the way we teach our core exercises. The key to understanding core training is realizing that the respiration process is not passive but active.

The first thing to understand about core training is that the diaphragm is, in fact, a muscle. And that muscle has as its antagonists the deep abdominal muscles that we seek to activate in our core training. Upon inhalation the dome-shaped diaphragm contracts concentrically and flattens, much like a group of children at camp pulling down on a parachute. On exhalation, specifically late in a maximal exhalation, the deep abdominals contract concentrically, effectively pushing the diaphragm back up into its dome shape. With proper breathing we have an interplay of eccentric and concentric contractions of the diaphragm and deep abdominals.

Mullin reinforced this concept in an article entitled "The Value of Blowing Up a Balloon" (Boyle, Olinick, and Lewis 2010). The article describes the action of blowing up a balloon without taking the balloon out of the mouth. What occurs is a process of nasal inhalation and aggressive mouth exhalation. With each exhale the deep abdominals are forced to work harder and harder against the elastic energy of the balloon. By the time the balloon is ready to pop, the connection between the abdominals and exhalation has been solidly reinforced. What we used to call a draw-in can actually be viewed as the maximal concentric contraction portion of proper maximal exhalation.

So now breathing is an integral part of our core training. Indeed, every core exercise essentially revolves around breathing. We eliminated time and count breaths in an attempt to get our athletes and clients to lengthen both their inhalation and exhalation to get proper muscular synergy.

CORE TRAINING PROGRESSION IN THE WEEKLY PROGRAM

Progressing core work is simple. Three sets of 8 to 12 repetitions are done initially for exercises that utilize weights. Stabilization exercises generally start with three sets of 25 seconds done in five sets of 5-second holds. Physical therapist Al Visnick introduced this concept to me with the statement: "If you want to train the stabilizers, you have to give them time to stabilize." One-second holds cannot work the stabilizers as effectively as a 5-second contraction. You can use time instead of reps to determine the length of a set. Five reps take approximately 30 to 60 seconds. These are general guidelines and can be adjusted based on the athlete's age and experience.

For any exercise using body weight, progress over a three-week period as follows:

Week 1: 3 × 8

Week 2: 3 × 10

Week 3: 3 × 12

After week 3, progress to a slightly more difficult version of the exercise (usually denoted as progression 1), reduce the number of repetitions, and again follow the same progression.

Remember that core work must be taught and coached like any other portion of a program. Simply doing core work at the beginning of the strength program rather than leaving it until the end is not enough. Coaches should teach core work as well as or better than any other facet of the program. A properly taught core training program aids in injury reduction, strength improvement, and speed improvement by increasing the ability to maintain trunk position in strength exercises, jumps, and sprints. In addition, a well-designed torso program can markedly improve performance in striking sports. These benefits cannot be overstated.

Antiextension Progression

Developing the ability of the anterior core to prevent extension of the lumbar spine (and the resultant accompanying anterior pelvic tilt) may be the most critical part of core training and most certainly should be the starting point for the core program. With anterior pelvic tilt and lower crossed syndrome, the anterior core muscles are unable to control extension of the spine and anterior rotation of the pelvis. In the past a combination of stretching and strengthening was often recommended, but the obvious step of working the anterior abdominals to prevent extension of the lumbar spine and the accompanying anterior tilt was not recognized. Current concepts now tell us to train these muscles to prevent extension and to stabilize the pelvis. I like to teach both the plank and the stability ball rollout in phase 1 to every athlete, hence the 1A and 1B designations in the exercises.

FRONT PLANK
BASELINE 1A

Every athlete should learn how to hold a perfect plank (see figure 7.5) for 30 seconds. (I am not a fan of planks beyond 30 seconds. Long-duration planks are both unnecessary and boring.)

1. Start on the elbows and forearms. Begin with 15-second holds, thinking about one long 15-second exhale. This will really fire up the deep abdominal muscles. (Don't be surprised if 10-second exhales are tough.)

2. Remember a perfect plank looks like a person who is standing. It's not a prone isometric crunch. The pelvis should be neutral or normal. In other words, do not move into a large posterior tilt via a big rectus abdominis contraction.

3. Squeeze everything. Push the floor with the forearms, squeeze the glutes, and tighten the quads and the deep abdominals.

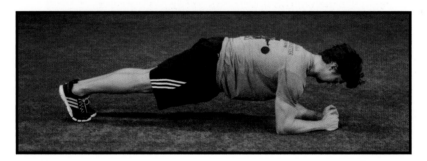

Figure 7.5   Front plank.

TORSO-ELEVATED FRONT PLANK
REGRESSION 1

If your athletes or clients can't hold a good front plank, simply use physics to your advantage and reduce their relative weight by inclining them. Try starting with elbows and forearms on a standard exercise bench.

⊳ STABILITY BALL ROLLOUT
BASELINE 1B

The stability ball rollout (see figure 7.6) is really just a short lever (kneeling) plank in which the lever arm is lengthened and shortened by rolling the ball away. Visualize the stability ball like a big ab wheel. The weaker the athlete, the bigger the ball should be to start. Stability balls come in centimeter sizes; 65 and 75 cm balls are good for beginners. It is essential that *everyone* start the antiextension progression with a combination of stability ball rollouts and front planks. Even athletes who have strong abs (or think they do) should do stability ball rollouts twice a week for the first three weeks. Starting with a wheel increases the chance of straining the abdominal muscles or hurting the back.

1. Begin in tall kneeling with the glutes and abs tight. Hands are on the ball.
2. Exhale while rolling forward, moving from hands to elbows. Stay in the tall kneeling position, tight from the top of the head to the knees.
3. Think about squeezing the glutes to keep the hips extended and exhaling to tighten the core and keep the spine stable. The key is that the core (the spine from hips to head) does not move into extension.

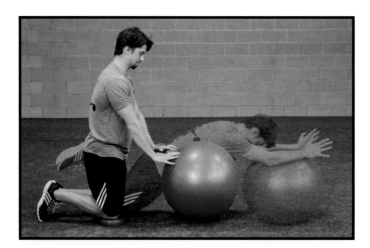

Figure 7.6   Stability ball rollout.

⊳ BODY SAW
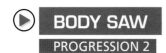
PROGRESSION 2

The body saw (see figure 7.7) is similar to the stability ball rollout in that it is a plank with a lengthening and shortening lever arm. In the body saw, the athlete begins in a plank position with the feet either on a slide-board surface or on two Valslides. Instead of pushing down into the floor, the action is like that of a saw, with a forward and back action coming from the shoulders. As the shoulders move into flexion, the lever arm is lengthened and the anterior core stress is increased.

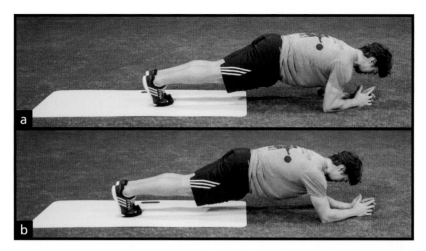

Figure 7.7   Body saw.

1. Think of the body saw as a plank with motion. The body should remain rigid from head to heels.

2. Go only as far as necessary to feel an increased stress on the anterior core. If it is felt in the back, the range of motion is too great.

3. The key to adding motion is to add a greater core stability challenge. It's not how far an athlete can go, it's how far he needs to go to create an increased core challenge.

Body saws move from time to reps. Follow the body-weight progression of 8-10-12.

AB DOLLY
PROGRESSION 3

I know, an infomercial piece of equipment. Ab Dollies are a bit pricey, but they make the transition from the stability ball to the ab wheel much easier. It's a physics thing. The Ab Dolly allows the user to be on the elbows first to get a short lever version of the ab wheel rollout (see figure 7.8).

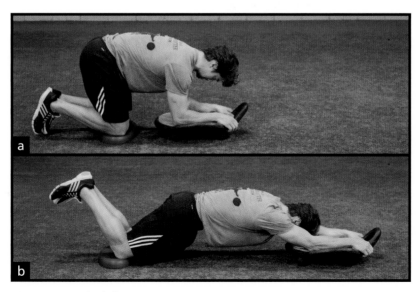

Figure 7.8   Ab dolly.

▶ AB WHEEL ROLLOUT
PROGRESSION 4

An Ab Dolly can be substituted for a wheel in this exercise. Simply grasp the sides of the Ab Dolly with the hands to lengthen the lever. I like the wheel better because you get better diagonals when you get more advanced, but for phase 3 it really doesn't matter. The key is that the moving piece is now a full arm's length away. Ab wheel rollouts (see figure 7.9) are an advanced core exercise. Starting with ab wheel rollouts can cause an abdominal strain, so make sure to follow the progression sequence.

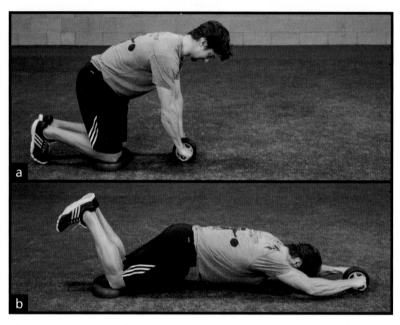

Figure 7.9   Ab wheel rollout.

VALSLIDE OR SLIDE-BOARD ROLLOUTS
PROGRESSION 5

The Valslide or slide board adds a frictional component. Instead of the wheel rolling, body weight creates drag. This makes the exercise harder, particularly the concentric, or return, portion. The athlete has to pull herself back in.

Antirotation Exercises

Antirotation is the new trend in core training. When you think of antirotation, think of a force being delivered that is trying to cause trunk rotation, and the athlete's job is to prevent that from happening. As we mentioned earlier, that is the real job of the rotary muscles of the core.

There are two categories of antirotation exercises. The first group is progressions of the plank that move from what we would call a four-point position (two elbows or two hands and two feet) to a three-point position (generally one elbow or hand and two feet). These are three-point versions of the plank. The second category of antirotation exercises is best described as diagonal patterns. Forces are introduced at various angles, and the core muscles must counter these forces in their antirotary function. This antirotation category includes exercises such as chops, lifts, press-outs, and push–pulls. These are stability exercises. Early attempts at rotary exercises included flawed activities such as wood choppers. Many early attempts at rotational core work were completely off base and were simply hip flexion patterns done in a diagonal.

Antirotation Plank Progressions

Any time an arm or leg is moved, a front plank moves from an antiextension exercise to an antirotation exercise. For this reason our plank progressions are under the antirotation category. Please note: All our plank antirotation progressions are arm reaches or movements. I am not a fan of leg lifts as plank progressions because I think the significant weight of the lower limbs makes these difficult to do safely.

PLANK REACH
PROGRESSION 1

The plank reach (see figure 7.10) is the simplest progression from the antiextension front plank to the antirotation category. In a plank reach the athlete is simply asked to reach for an object in front of him. We generally use a cone placed approximately 12 inches (30 cm) away. The athlete is still in a position on the forearms and elbows. The key to the plank reach is the maintenance of core stability. The athlete must continue to hold a perfect plank position while reaching. Everything should continue to look just like the plank as the athlete transitions from four-point support to three-point support. The three-point support position produces a diagonal force across the core that must be countered to prevent movement.

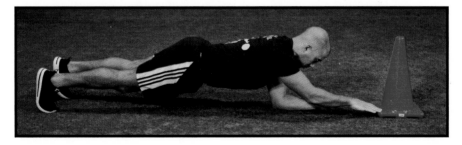

Figure 7.10   Plank reach.

CLOCK PLANK
PROGRESSION 2

The clock plank is similar to the plank reach but the athlete is on the hands instead of the elbows (see figure 7.11). Instead of simply reaching forward, the athlete moves the right hand to 12 o'clock and then the left hand to 12 o'clock. The right hand then moves to 1 while the left moves to the 11 o'clock position. This continues around the imaginary clock face, with the hands making seven touches on each side. Clock planks can be done in any number of ways, using 12 to 6 as 1 set or doing 12 to 6 to 12 to increase difficulty. Again the key is core and scapular stability in the presence of diagonal rotational forces.

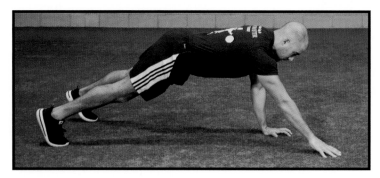

Figure 7.11   Clock plank.

PLANK ROW
PROGRESSION 3

In the plank row (see figure 7.12) the athlete is again in an elbow-extended position but has a set of dumbbells in the hands. The action changes from reaching to rowing. Plank rows have numerous names and variations, but all should be seen as antirotation core exercises, not strength exercises or a circus act. My recommendation is to use hex dumbbells that don't roll and to never use kettlebells. The risk of wrist injury far outweighs any potential benefit.

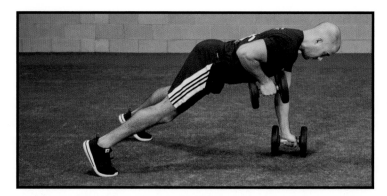

Figure 7.12   Plank row.

Antilateral Flexion

In the same way that we want to see the anterior core assume the role of antiextension, we want to see the lateral muscles also assume the role of stabilizers. In the past, exercises such as side bends have been used to train the lateral flexion capability of the core. However, we now see that all of the core muscles prevent motion more than cause it. The lateral flexors (primary obliques and quadratus lumborum) actually act to prevent the core from collapsing into lateral flexion.

SIDE PLANK
BASELINE

The side plank is the lateral version of the front plank and is the best place to begin to incorporate the idea of antilateral flexion. All your athletes and clients should learn how to hold a perfect side plank for 30 seconds.

1. Start on the elbow with the shoulder blade pulled down and back. Begin with 15-second holds, thinking about one, big, long 15-second exhale. This will really cause you to fire the deep abdominal muscles. (Don't be surprised if 10-second exhales are tough.)
2. The perfect side plank looks like what the person would look like if they were going to be shot out of a cannon. Think long and straight. I like to extend and hold the opposite arm.
3. Squeeze everything. Squeeze the glutes and tighten the quads and the deep abdominals.

SHORT-LEVER SIDE PLANK
REGRESSION 1

To regress the side plank, all you need to do is shorten the lever by bending the knees.

SIDE PLANK ROW
PROGRESSION 1

A simple way to progress the side plank is to add a row with a band or off a cable column. Basically, this adds a transverse plane stress to what is initially frontal plane stability. Think of the row as a fairly light exercise basically incorporated to increase the concentration need in the plank. Instead of time, now do repetitions of the row following our 8-10-12 progression.

SUITCASE CARRY
PROGRESSION 2

The suitcase carry is basically a walk holding a single dumbbell or kettlebell in one hand. The key to the suitcase carry is that it is actually a loaded dynamic version of the side plank. I can recall sitting in a Stuart McGill lecture and having the ah-ha moment of an exercise I didn't truly understand becoming an exercise that I understood and appreciated. I can remember seeing many of the loaded carries used in Strongman events and thinking of them as foolish. Now I see myself as foolish. Progression here can be distance travelled, load, or any combination of the two.

FARMER'S WALK
PROGRESSION 3

The farmer's walk is a progression from the suitcase carry, but actually it shifts from a core exercise to a hip exercise. The addition of a balanced load in each hand makes the exercise potentially less of an antilateral flexion exercise and more of a challenge to the hip stabilizers. McGill has also noted in his lectures that the greatest hip loads he recorded have been in Strongman loaded carry events such as the Yoke Walk. In any case, all loaded carries fall in the core training category.

Chop and Lift Patterns and Progressions

Physical therapist Gray Cook first introduced the chop and lift patterns in the late 1990s, basing them on the PNF diagonal concepts of Knott and Voss. Cook's article "Functional Training for the Torso" (1997) took these diagonal concepts from the rehab world and developed an entirely new classification of exercises.

Cook advocated diagonal patterns from high to low (chop) and from low to high (lift) to develop core stability against dynamic forces. In the chop and lift variations, the arms transfer force on a diagonal plane through a relatively stable torso. The exercises presented here have been modified from Cook's original concepts. Any rotation in these exercises should come from turning the shoulders.

For all the chop and lift exercises, do three sets of 10 and increase the weight in week 2, or use a set weight and an 8-10-12 progression.

HALF-KNEELING IN-LINE STABLE CHOP
PROGRESSION 1A

Progression 1A begins in the half-kneeling position with the feet in line. This means the front foot, back knee, and back foot are all in a straight line. This narrow base of support forces the athlete to learn the proper mechanics and is done intentionally to require the use of light loads. We use small rubber balance beams to create our in-line position, but a two- by four-inch (5 by 10 cm) board can work just as well. The beam or board should be positioned approximately two to three feet (.6 to .9 m) away from the cable column to create the proper diagonal.

At MBSC we use a triceps rope handle held with a thumb-up grip for both chops and lifts. We teach the chop as a pull to the chest followed by a press away. The movement presents like a pull-down combined

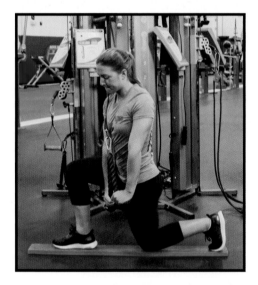

Figure 7.13   Half-kneeling in-line stable chop.

with a triceps press-down done on a diagonal across the body (see figure 7.13). Teach this as a distinct two-part action, a pull and a push. It is also important that in diagonal patterns the eyes follow the hands. Looking at the hands creates the ideal amount of control over thoracic rotation.

There are two keys to the half-kneeling chop. The first is the core stability and balance necessary to move the load diagonally from high to low. The second is the antirotational strength to resist being pulled back toward the weight stack on the eccentric portion of the lift. The athlete must have sagittal-plane stability on the beam while controlling a force moving through the frontal plane. In addition, the athlete must stabilize in both the frontal and transverse planes. The key action here is firing the glutes on the down (outside) leg to stabilize the hip and core. The concept of antirotation is based on stabilizing against rotational forces rather than producing rotation. Sahrmann (2002) states: "During most daily activities the role of the abdominal muscles is to provide isometric support and to limit the degree of rotation of the trunk. . . . a large percentage of low back problems occur because the abdominal muscles are not maintaining tight control over the pelvis and the spine at the L5-S1 level" (71). Antirotation provides the tight control Sahrmann refers to.

EXOS founder Mark Verstegen probably deserves credit for moving Cook's rehab thoughts into the performance world and making rotary training a part of the training vocabulary.

1. Inside knee is up. Outside knee is down.
2. Front foot, back hip, and back foot are in line.
3. Action is a pull down to the chest followed by a press away.

HALF-KNEELING IN-LINE STABLE LIFT
PROGRESSION 1B

Think of the lift as the opposite of the chop. Lift patterns are diagonals from low to high and are progressed in much the same manner as chops. Progression 1B uses the same in-line position as the chop, except in the lift pattern the outside knee is up and the inside knee is down (see figure 7.14). The action is now a pull to the chest followed by a diagonal pushing action. The same triceps rope setup is used as in the chop pattern.

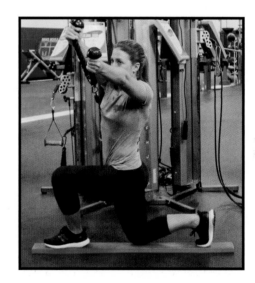

Figure 7.14   Half-kneeling in-line stable lift.

1. Inside knee is down. Outside knee is up.
2. Feet, hip, and knees are in line.
3. Action is a pull to the chest followed by a diagonal press away.

▶ LUNGE-POSITION CHOP
PROGRESSION 2A

The second progression is a simple yet difficult change. The back knee is now lifted off the ground or beam, and the athlete must hold a static lunge posture while performing the chopping action (see figure 7.15). Again, loads are light and the exercise is a controlled pull–push movement. This remains very much a core stability exercise.

These progressions are based on Cook's concepts of moving from kneeling to a split stance (lunge) to standing and eventually to a single leg and are based on Cook's observation that the best way to simplify an exercise is to limit the number of joints involved. In kneeling it is very easy to focus on the hips and core because the knees are to a great extent eliminated from the focus of the exercise. Lunge position provides an increased stability challenge from the half-kneeling position by decreasing the number of stable points in contact with the ground from three (foot, knee, foot) to two feet. Eliminating the knee joint as a stable point provides an additional stability challenge to the core.

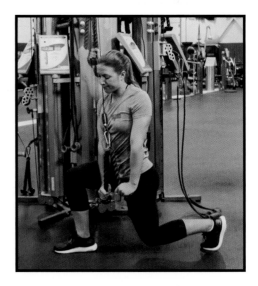

Figure 7.15   Lunge-position chop.

1. Back knee is one to two inches (2.5 to 5 cm) off the floor.
2. Inside knee is up, outside is down as in a split-squat hold.
3. Upper body action remains unchanged and still features a controlled pull–push or pull–press.

LUNGE-POSITION LIFT
PROGRESSION 2B

This exercise is identical to the in-line version except the back knee is lifted off the ground or beam. All other aspects remain the same.

1. Inside knee is down, outside is up as in a split-squat hold.
2. Upper body action is a controlled pull to the chest with a press away.

STANDING CHOP ▶
PROGRESSION 3A

The standing chop (see figure 7.16) is a very different exercise. The push–pull action becomes one smooth, fluid, explosive movement. Unlike the previous two versions, the foot position moves from a split stance to the feet parallel. In phase 3 the diagonal patterns cease to be stability exercises and become dynamic rotational power exercises. I like to have my athletes visualize grabbing an object and throwing it aggressively to the ground with the same pull–push pattern used in the in-line and lunge versions. In truth, we have moved from antirotation to explosive rotation.

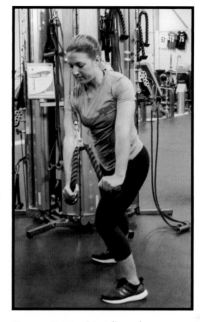

Figure 7.16   Standing chop.

STANDING LIFT ▶
PROGRESSION 3B

The standing lift pattern (see figure 7.17) is what EXOS president Mark Verstegen once described as a diagonal push–press. The motion is an explosive cross-body squat to stand finishing with the arms extended on the side opposite the cable column. We do not coach rotation but rather simply coach a squat to stand action. The rotation comes naturally because of the combination of the parallel foot placement and the load position.

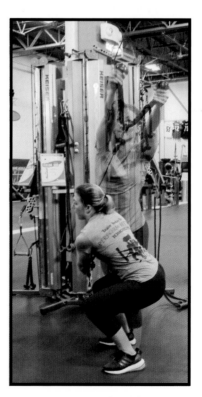

Figure 7.17   Standing lift.

▶ STANDING TRANSVERSE CHOP
PROGRESSION 3C

The transverse chop (see figure 7.18) is a great exercise for hitting and striking athletes and is something we have added to our exercise menu the past few years. The exercise is still done in a pull–push pattern and from a parallel stance as in the previous two exercises. The triceps rope is held with thumbs pointing toward the cable column. This is extremely important to make the exercise feel smooth and to take pressure off the wrists.

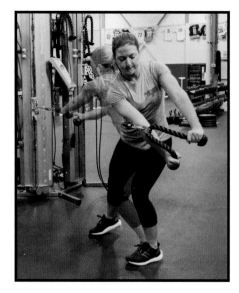

Figure 7.18   Standing transverse chop.

▶ STEP-UP LIFT
PROGRESSION 4

The step-up lift (see figure 7.19) might be the most functional of the diagonal patterns because it incorporates unilateral lower body exercise with multiplanar upper body actions. In the step-up lift the inside foot is placed on a 12-inch (30 cm) plyo box, and instead of a squat to stand pattern, a step-up to stand pattern is used. All upper body actions remain the same, but the lower pattern now becomes unilateral support in the extended position. This exercise creates a great diagonal connection between the glutes, pelvic stabilizers, and upper body muscles.

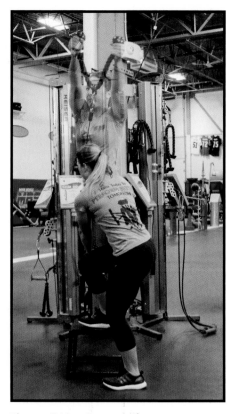

Figure 7.19   Step-up lift.

BRIDGING YOUR WAY TO HEALTHY HAMSTRINGS

The bridging exercises are included in the core chapter but might also be featured in the section under activation or mobility. Bridging exercises and quadruped exercises can be viewed as core exercises, as motor control exercises, or as activation exercises. In any case, they should be done initially as part of the warm-up and then eventually morph into exercises such as slide-board leg curls.

COOK HIP LIFT
BASELINE 1

This baseline exercise places dual emphasis on the glutes and the core muscles. The Cook hip lift (see figure 7.20) develops glute and hamstring strength, but more importantly, it teaches the critical difference between hip motion and lumbar spine motion—an important goal of all the bridging and quadruped exercises. In many exercises that target the hamstrings and glutes, it is easy to mistakenly use more range of motion at the lumbar spine than at the hip. This teaches the athlete to arch the back instead of extend the hip.

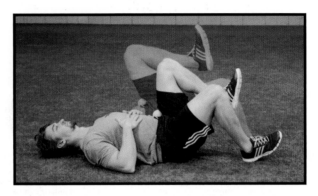

Figure 7.20   Cook hip lift.

To perform the Cook hip lift, lie on the back with both feet flat on the floor. From the start position pull one knee tightly to the chest with both arms to limit movement at the lumbar spine. To ensure that the knee stays tight against the chest, place a tennis ball near the bottom of the rib cage and pull the thigh up to hold the ball in place. The ball must not fall out during the set. The opposite knee is bent 90 degrees, and the foot on the floor is dorsiflexed. Extend the hip by pushing the heel down into the floor. Pushing though the heel encourages posterior chain use and prevents the athlete from pushing with the quads. Keep the toes up. Last key is to cue a big exhale on the concentric contraction. Think inhale through the nose and exhale hard through the mouth for the entire 5-second isometric hold.

Don't be surprised if the range of motion is limited initially to a few degrees. This exercise has two purposes:

1. It teaches the difference between range of motion of the hip and range of motion of the lumbar spine.

2. It develops additional flexibility in the psoas because of the reciprocal nature of the exercise. It's impossible to contract the glutes and hamstrings on one side without relaxing the psoas on the opposite side.

Perform five 5-second holds on each side and progress by adding one per week.

HANDS-FREE COOK HIP LIFT
PROGRESSION 1

The first progression is to use the hip flexors on the flexed-hip side to hold the tennis ball. This adds complexity to the exercise because the athlete now has to contract flexors on one side and extensors on the other.

Stay with the same five times 5-second-hold format.

DOUBLE-LEG BRIDGE
BASELINE 2

This is another baseline exercise that requires the athlete to transfer the knowledge gained about hip range of motion from the Cook hip lift. Begin again in a hook-lying position with both heels down and toes up (dorsiflexed), and raise the hips to create a straight line from the knee through the hip to the shoulder (see

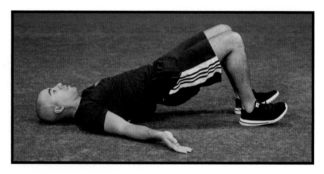

Figure 7.21　Double-leg bridge.

figure 7.21). Create and maintain this posture by using the glutes and hamstrings, not by extending the lumbar spine. Any drop in the hips drastically reduces the effectiveness of the exercise. At the top point, exhale maximally to draw in the abdominals. Maintain this top position for a 5-second exhale.

Before attempting this exercise, it is important to learn the difference between hip movement and lumbar spine movement through an exercise such as the Cook hip lift. Most athletes who do not understand this distinction arch the back to attempt to extend the hips.

Do five 5-second holds to complete one set. Add one more rep per week.

BRIDGE WITH ALTERNATE MARCH
PROGRESSION 1

The next step in the progression is to add a small alternate march to the isometric bridge. Simply alternate lifting one foot and then the other off the ground. Do not let the opposite hip drop when the foot is lifted. This progression targets the hip rotators and multifidus because of the rotational stress applied to the spinal column as a result of moving from four support points (shoulders and

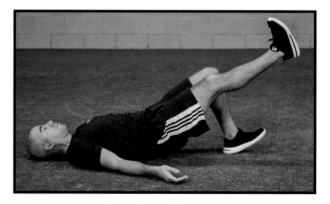

Figure 7.22　Bridge with alternate march.

feet) to three support points (shoulders and one foot). Push down through the heel and activate the glutes on the same side as the supporting foot. See figure 7.22.

For marches do sets of 8-10-12 each side

Quadruped Progression

The quadruped exercises are frequently viewed as rehabilitative and have largely been ignored by strength and conditioning coaches and athletic trainers, possibly because of the old theory that strong abs equate to a healthy back. Like the supine progression, the quadruped exercises may not make sense at first glance, but only because they are often performed incorrectly. In many cases the results of these exercises become the opposite of what was intended.

Quadruped exercises should teach athletes how to recruit the glutes and hamstrings while maintaining a stable torso. Instead, athletes often learn that they can mimic hip extension by extending (or hyperextending) the lumbar spine. The purpose of the quadruped progression is to teach the athlete to stabilize the core with the deep abdominals and multifidus muscles and to simultaneously use the hip extensors to extend the hip. A great deal of low back pain is related to poor function of the hip that must be compensated for by lumbar extension or lumbar rotation.

QUADRUPED HIP EXTENSION ON ELBOWS

BASELINE

The beginning point for the quadruped progression has the athlete on the elbows and knees instead of the hands and knees (see figure 7.23). This automatically creates a greater degree of hip flexion, closing the angle between the hip and trunk from 90 degrees down to 45 degrees. The result is less ability to extend the lumbar spine. The athlete is in effect forced into using the hip extensors to a greater degree.

In this exercise the hip is extended with the knee bent. This flexed-knee position creates

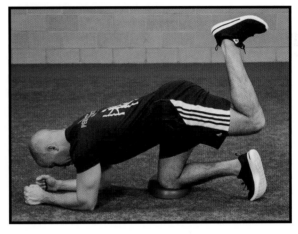

Figure 7.23   Quadruped hip extension on elbows.

a poor length–tension relationship for the hamstrings and again forces the glutes to be the primary hip extensor. Effectively, by correct positioning we have decreased the ability of the lumbar spine to extend and act as a hip extensor, and we have decreased the ability of the hamstrings to compensate for a weak or underactive glute.

Do 5 × 5 seconds, with a big exhale on the concentric contraction. Progress to 6 × 5 seconds and 7 × 5 seconds.

QUADRUPED HIP EXTENSION

PROGRESSION 1

Progress from being on the elbows to being on the hands with the elbows extended. This exercise can be done with bent legs or as a hip and knee extension. For the straight-leg version, it is key that the toes remain dorsiflexed and the foot come up no higher than the butt. The hip extension should be a straight-out "heel to the wall" action. This version is most often done with too much lumbar movement. Think core stability. If the heel stays level with the butt, the back cannot extend.

Do 5 × 5 seconds, with a big exhale on the concentric contraction. Progress to 6 × 5 seconds and 7 × 5 seconds.

QUADRUPED ALTERNATING ARM AND LEG
PROGRESSION 2

Now add an alternating arm and leg action to the quadruped hip extension (see figure 7.24). This is an advanced exercise that is often done poorly by beginners. Remember that when these exercises are done incorrectly, they are potentially damaging because they reinforce the pattern of lumbar extension for hip extension that we are trying to eliminate.

Do 5 × 5 seconds, with a big exhale on the concentric contraction. Progress to 6 × 5 seconds and 7 × 5 seconds.

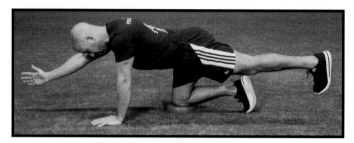

Figure 7.24   Quadruped alternating arm and leg.

Get-Ups and Sit-Ups

Although we emphasize doing core exercises primarily for stability, there are two exercises we incorporate that might be considered in the more conventional category: the Turkish get-up (we just use the term *get-up*) and the straight-leg sit-up. Both exercises involve some element of trunk flexion, but the low repetitions make them both beneficial and relatively safe. We caution against crunches and conventional bent-leg sit-ups but still incorporate the get-up and the straight-leg sit-up.

STRAIGHT-LEG SIT-UP

The straight-leg sit-up (see figure 7.25) is exactly what it says and is actually a very difficult core exercise that is best done for low reps. We never exceed sets of 10. The straight-leg sit-up involves a small amount of trunk flexion and a large amount of hip flexion. Some of the old wives' tales of fitness have cautioned against straight-leg sit-ups, but the reality is there is no good reason to avoid them. The key is a slow ascent and a slow descent. If momentum is needed to complete a rep, then the athlete is not ready for this exercise.

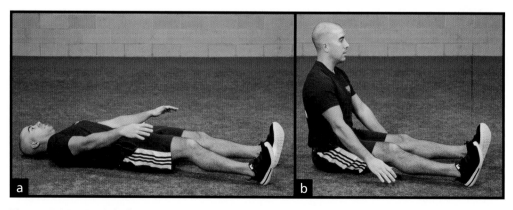

Figure 7.25   Straight-leg sit-up.

Progression is very simple. Begin with the arms at the side to control the length of the lever arm. Think squeezing up and lowering down. There should be no rocking or momentum. To progress, move the hands across the chest and eventually add a plate in the extended arms. Do two or three sets of 10 reps.

GET-UP ▶

Five years ago I would have told you this exercise was foolish. My, how things change. An old quote says that "when the student is ready, the teacher appears." I know this is true for me. The teachers in my case were a client and Gray Cook.

I had heard Gray Cook praise get-ups for a few years and wondered why he had started to become a kettlebell enthusiast. The epiphany for me came not through Gray but through a 60-year-old client. My client had difficulty getting up from the floor. The process often looked painful and uncoordinated. I was often tempted to help him up but resisted, as it seemed necessary for him to learn. One day as we both stretched, I thought through my actions and his. My client struggled on all fours to get up, sometimes moving from a deep squat. I on the other hand seemed to bounce right up. I attempted to explain to my client how I did this. I said, "Roll onto your elbow and then up to your hand. Then get up on one knee." Suddenly it hit me: I was teaching him how to "get-up." In a flash the Turkish get-up went from a silly YouTube feat of strength into a basic primal motor pattern. The get-up in its simplest sense is how we get up from the floor. Oh, how I hate those aha moments that make me feel foolish. Now everyone works on get-ups just like they do squats.

We do our get-ups progressively because they take some time to learn. Although the purists will be horrified, the get-up is basically a loaded variation of the straight-leg sit-up and involves some of the elements of the phenomenon of rolling that is now so popular.

The Get-Up Setup

Volumes of both written and video information are available on how to do the get-up. In simple terms, the athlete lies on the back with the kettlebell at the end of one extended arm. The same-side leg is bent with the foot flat on the floor. The opposite leg is straight and abducted about 20 to 30 degrees.

QUARTER GET-UP
BASELINE

The quarter get-up (see figure 7.26a) is simply a roll to the elbow opposite the kettlebell. The elbow drives down hard into the floor as the kettlebell is driven toward the ceiling. Think rotational sit-up. In phase 1, that is all we do for three or four reps each side.

HALF GET-UP
PROGRESSION 1

In the half get-up (see figure 7.26b) the athlete moves from elbow to hand and then to a bridge. Effectively, the action is a straight-leg bridge opposite the kettlebell and a bent-leg bridge or hip lift on the same side as the kettlebell.

FULL GET-UP
PROGRESSION 2

From the bridge the athlete moves to a half kneel and then stands (see figure 7.26c). To get back, the process is simply reversed. The DVD *Kettlebells From the Ground Up* (Cook and Jones 2010) is a great teaching resource for the get-up.

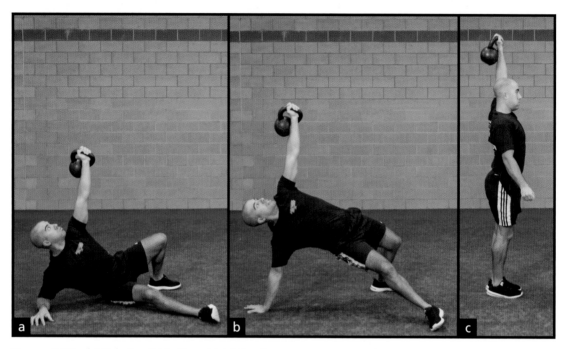

Figure 7.26　(a) Quarter, (b) half, and (c) full get-ups.

MEDICINE BALL TRAINING

The medicine ball may be the simplest and safest tool for developing total-body power, rotary power and, anterior-core power. In fact, the medicine ball has become a staple in just about every functional training program.

The key to medicine ball training is the ability to develop power in hip internal and external rotation and to move that power from the ground through the core. Many coaches have mistakenly attempted to develop core power with weights using exercises that focus on lumbar rotation. This is a potentially dangerous mistake that can lead to back injury. Rotary power lies in the hips and not in the core. As discussed previously, lumbar rotation is potentially dangerous and not at all functional. Hip rotation on the other hand is not only functional but safe.

Many athletes mistakenly think that rotary power means lumbar rotation and must be shown that many of the movements previously viewed as lumbar rotation are actually hip rotation. Movements such as the golf swing, the baseball swing, and just about any striking or throwing skill are accomplished with hip movement and a relatively stable lumbar spine.

Many of these medicine ball drills can be viewed as multipurpose and multifunction. Overhead throws can be used to train the anterior core for power but are also vital for throwing athletes to work on the decelerative capability of the posterior shoulder musculature. Rotational throws develop the power in the hip necessary to strike objects, while chest throws develop power in the pushing muscles.

The medicine ball is a safe, adaptable, and effective tool for developing hip and core power. Medicine ball training is best viewed in the same way that Olympic lifting and plyometrics are considered for the core and hips. Most of the core exercises previously described in this chapter address core stability and strength. Medicine ball training converts all the strength and stability developed through other core exercises into usable power. Most importantly, proper medicine ball progressions develop explosive power both safely and effectively.

Again, credit for many of these concepts should go to Mark Verstegen of EXOS, who heavily influenced my thinking on the subject of medicine ball training beginning in the 1990s. Before meeting Mark and watching his athletes train, I had never envisioned a solid concrete wall to throw medicine balls against as a requirement for a facility. Now, nearly 20 years later, I could not imagine designing a facility that did not include a medicine ball wall.

Medicine ball training is far superior when done against a wall. A partner is a poor substitute because the athlete cannot throw with maximum power. In any case, masonry wall space is now a basic requirement for a medicine ball program and for a well-designed facility.

Medicine ball throws are critical for all clients but may be most important for our adult clients. Adults are losing power at a rate of almost 1.5 times the rate they lose strength. In other words, a client who loses 10 percent of her strength loses 15 percent of her power.

A good set of throws mimics a good series of shots or swings and should be fluid, with explosive concentric contractions. For standing throws, athletes should stand approximately a body length away from the wall and throw as if they want to damage both the wall and the ball. Athletes can move closer to or farther from the wall, depending on their power output.

Proper ball selection is vital. Most strength athletes believe that heavier is better in all things. With the medicine ball, this is certainly not the case.

Any time an athlete struggles to throw a medicine ball, the ball is too heavy or potentially too large. The guidelines for medicine ball weight in table 7.1 are based on our experience with thousands of athletes. For beginners, a lighter ball works better. For smaller athletes, a smaller diameter works better. If you have any doubts about ball weight, go down 2 pounds or 1 kilogram. Initially all medicine balls were available only in kilograms; however, the rapid acceptance of medicine balls in the United States has resulted in balls now being manufactured in both pounds and kilograms.

For overhead throws for baseball players, we stay at 4 pounds (2 kg).

The key to medicine ball training is velocity. Emphasize speed of movement, not ball weight. And always remember this simple rule: If it looks too heavy, it probably is.

Table 7.1   Guidelines for Medicine Ball Selection

Athlete's weight	Ball weight (rotation)	Ball weight (overhead)
100-135 lb (45-61 kg)	4 lb (2 kg)	2 lb (1 kg)
135-175 lb (61-79 kg)	6 lb (3 kg)	4 lb (2 kg)
175-200 lb (79-90 kg)	8 lb (4 kg)	6 lb (3 kg)
200-250 lb (90-113 kg)	10 lb (5 kg)	8 lb (4 kg)

Advantages of Medicine Ball Training

- The medicine ball allows the user to work in a sports-general position or pattern. These patterns are similar to the golf swing, tennis swing, baseball swing, and numerous other striking skills.
- Medicine balls bridge the gap from conventional strength and endurance exercises for the core to power development through the core. Think of medicine ball work as plyometrics for the core stabilizers and hip rotators. The medicine ball allows the muscles to contract at speeds similar to that encountered in sports.
- The medicine ball teaches summation of force, from the ground through the legs, through the core, and finally out through the arms. This transfer process is the essence of core function. The athlete learns to transfer force from the ground to the ball, with the core as the vital link.
- Medicine ball training can be done alone if a concrete block wall is available.
- Working with the medicine ball also has a total-body conditioning effect.

Disadvantages of Medicine Ball Training

- You don't feel it. Athletes often judge core work by the burn. You do not feel the effect of medicine ball training until the next day.
- You need space. Medicine ball training takes up a large amount of space and requires masonry walls to throw against.
- You need many medicine balls in a range of sizes.

USING NONBOUNCING MEDICINE BALLS

I love the nonbouncing medicine balls, but I can't say I always did. You know the ones I mean—they look like the old-school leather balls your grandfather used in gym class. They are now covered in vinyl or Kevlar (or some fake leather), but they are still the same. They are relatively soft, and they don't bounce well.

About 10 years ago I bought some of these heavy, nonbouncing, vinyl-covered balls for performing upper body plyometrics. Primarily we used these balls for medicine ball bench presses. We would have one partner drop an 18- to 20-pound ball to an athlete lying on his back with arms extended, and the other athlete would throw the ball back. I really like this exercise for upper body power because it does not stress the shoulders like exercises such as plyometric push-ups do. The reason we used the nonbouncing balls is that they are softer and easier to handle when dropped.

A few years ago someone on my staff ordered some lighter nonbouncing balls for the younger athletes we train. The balls sat in the storage closet, and I wondered if we would ever use them. One day I took them all out. We had paid a lot of money for the balls, and I was trying to think of a good use for them. Just for the heck of it I threw one off the wall in a side-twist throw. Normally this throw is our standard rotational core and plyometric exercise, but the throw had always been done with a more conventional rubber medicine ball to get a plyometric effect.

My first thought was *These balls stink. They don't bounce back.* In response I threw the ball as hard as I could off the wall to get it to bounce back. It did, but weakly. Suddenly the lights came on. What I had initially perceived as a drawback to the nonbouncing ball suddenly became a huge positive. Think about this. Initially we had used rotational medicine ball throws for an explosive core exercise, a core plyo if you will. The fact that the balls bounced back allowed us to get a rhythmic pace and a plyometric effect. The ball coming off the wall forced us to use the core not only to accelerate the ball but also to create a deceleration and a switching effect. For years I thought that was such a great idea.

When I threw the light nonbouncing ball, I suddenly asked myself, *What are we doing rotational power exercises for?* I immediately answered my own question. The goal was shooting or hitting harder in sports such as baseball, ice hockey, field hockey, and golf. The next question I asked myself was *Is the eccentric component of the ball recoiling off the wall important?* The answer seemed to be no. The skill of striking seemed to be a 1 RM movement that was very powerful but was not repeated multiple times.

All of a sudden these light balls were not a mistake but a great new tool. We now actually use the nonbouncing balls for more of our throws than we use the rubber balls for. In fact, I think medicine ball slams and side throws are far better with the nonbouncing balls than with bouncing rubber ones. The exception to the rule might be overhead throws. Here we still focus on light rubber medicine balls. We position ourselves farther from the wall and catch the ball after one bounce.

If you have a medicine ball wall and like to use medicine ball throws in your program for core power, order a few nonbouncing balls. I like the 8-pound (4 kg) ball for most athletes. The balls now come in two diameters to accommodate smaller athletes. For kids, a 6-pound (3 kg) mini-ball works great.

In addition, the softer ball saves on fingers. We have sprained a few fingers and even broken one or two with our medicine ball throws. Yes, the nonbouncing balls are more expensive, but good tools are expensive. Try them. I think you'll like them.

Rotational Throws

Rotational throws are the best technique for developing power in the core and hip muscles. These exercises are particularly good for hockey, golf, tennis, baseball, and any other sport that requires explosive rotary action. Medicine ball throws develop hip power by teaching the athlete to better utilize hip internal and external rotation to draw power from the ground. The goal is not torso rotation but rather powerful hip rotation. The objective is to learn to transfer ground forces through a relatively stiff and stable core.

Much like some of our other core exercises, we progress from either tall kneeling or half kneeling to standing throws and eventually to stepping throws. The lunge position is difficult for medicine ball throws, so we often progress from a kneeling variation directly to a standing variation, skipping the lunge position.

Side-Throw Progressions

The side throw imitates a number of sports skills. These drills develop the explosive rotational torso strength so necessary for sports such as tennis, field hockey, ice hockey, lacrosse, and baseball. In side throws the emphasis should be on throwing from the hips.

A good side throw should look like a good swing or a good shot. Strive to develop a throwing style that has the appearance of the skill being improved. For a hockey player, for instance, the side throw should look like a slap shot; for a tennis player, it should look like a good swing. When teaching, draw on the athlete's or client's familiarity with the sport.

Perform 10 throws on the right side (see figure 7.27), then 10 throws on the left. Do three sets of 10 throws on each side for three weeks. Don't attempt to increase volume; throw harder and throw better. This is the progression for all rotational medicine ball work to follow.

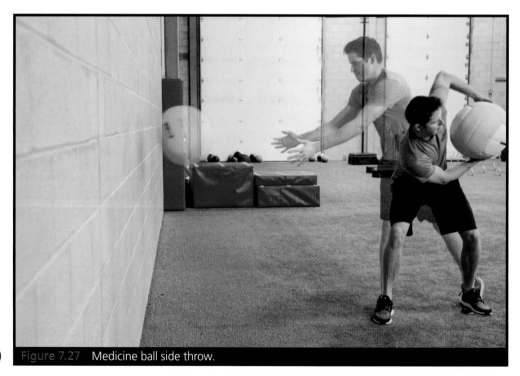

 Figure 7.27　Medicine ball side throw.

If medicine balls are for power, why do we do 10 reps? I might as well deal with this question right off the bat. Those fascinated with science will look at medicine ball throws, see 10-rep sets, and say, "That's not a power exercise." My answer is that science agrees with you but empiricism does not. We tried to follow science and do sets of five or six reps, but to be honest, it just didn't seem like enough. The load (ball weight) is light enough that 10 reps can be done with no loss of power or velocity.

HALF-KNEELING SIDE-TWIST THROW
PROGRESSION 1

As with our other core progressions, for most beginners we start with a half-kneeling version of the side-twist throw (see figure 7.28). This will be phase 1 in most of our athlete programs. As mentioned before, physical therapist Gray Cook popularized the idea of eliminating joints for teaching purposes. The half-kneeling position teaches hip rotation in the throws by effectively taking out the knees and ankles. By having the inside (closest to the wall) knee up, the athlete or client is forced to use the hips and the kneeling (back side) glute.

We teach a long-arm, long-lever throw with the inside hand under the ball and the outside hand behind the ball. Make sure this is a long-lever rotation and not a push. Encourage the mental link to a shot or swing to teach the use of the long lever arm, and watch for athletes reverting to more of a push. Also, make the clients aware it will feel awkward on their nondominant side.

1. Begin while half kneeling in a short lunge position, two to three feet (.6 to .9 m) from the wall; shoulders are perpendicular to the wall.

2. The arms are long, with the front hand under the ball and the back hand behind.

3. Think about throwing from the back knee and hip with some hip "pop."

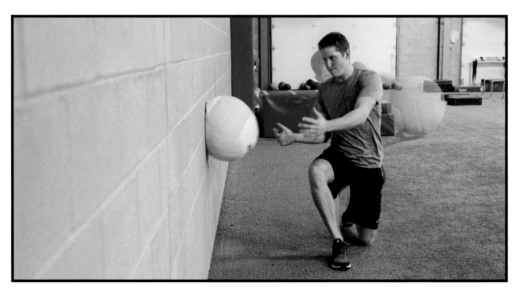

Figure 7.28   Medicine ball half-kneeling side-twist throw.

STANDING SIDE-TWIST THROW
PROGRESSION 2

As mentioned earlier, we skip the lunge-position throws for a very simple logistical reason. Our athletes and clients struggled to maintain the lunge position and to focus on the throw itself, so now we simply skip to standing. In certain cases we start younger or older athletes or clients immediately in standing (see figure 7.29). For high school and college athletes, we stick with a progression from half kneeling to standing to stepping, but with middle school kids and our adults, we begin in standing and simply say, "Throw the ball as hard as you can." This emphasis on a gross motor pattern often overcomes some technical hurdles. In much the same way, older clients may be too stiff through the hips and core to benefit from the half-kneeling position the way an athlete does and may also start in standing. Remember, progressions are fluid suggestions, not rigid rules.

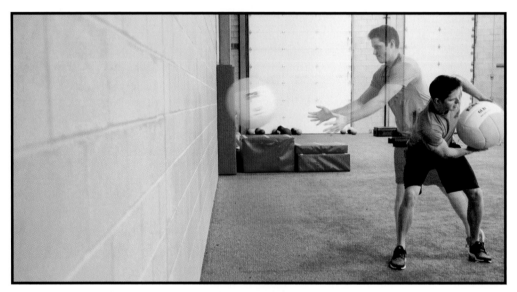

Figure 7.29   Medicine ball standing side-twist throw.

SIDE-TWIST THROW WITH STEP
PROGRESSION 3

The next step in the progression is to add movement to the throw. In progression 3, step toward the wall with the front foot to increase the force being generated from the back foot. Emphasis is on shifting weight from the back foot to the front. All other aspects of the side throw remain the same.

TWO-STEP SIDE-TWIST THROW
PROGRESSION 4

In our fourth progression, the athlete takes two steps toward the wall. Obviously the client or athlete now needs to be farther away from the wall. The two-step throw is more aggressive and violent and really mimics the actions of shooting on the move. The two-step throw also places greater stress on the front foot and hip.

Side-Throw Variations

Here are some side-throw variations athletes can work into their progressions.

FRONT-TWIST THROW
PROGRESSION 4

The front-twist throw (see figure 7.30) is another great general rotational exercise for the core. Front-twist throws are initially performed one side at a time. Again, teach the athlete or client to throw from the hips and feet and then through the trunk. Throw from the ground up with the hands as the final point. Face the wall with the body parallel to the wall. This basic defensive stance, with the knees bent and the hips down and back, is a fundamental sports-general stance and a simple starting point for any athlete. Front-twist throws are excellent for tennis players, who often hit from a perpendicular position, and for ice hockey players, who often shoot from a similar stance. Don't limit these throws to just these athletes, though; this drill can be beneficial for any client.

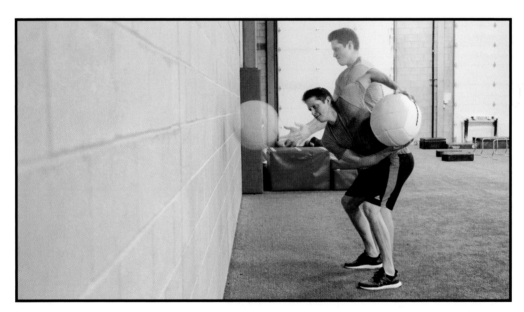

Figure 7.30   Medicine ball front-twist throw.

ALTERNATING FRONT-TWIST THROW
PROGRESSION 5

In the alternating front-twist throw, instead of performing 10 throws from one side and then 10 from the other, the athlete alternates sides for 20 throws. The side-to-side movement should be fluid and athletic. This exercise demands slightly more coordination and athleticism.

⏵ SINGLE-LEG FRONT-TWIST THROW
PROGRESSION 6

This advanced exercise adds difficulty as well as great proprioceptive stimulus for the ankle, knee, and hip. It requires a higher level of balance and coordination and heavily involves the hip rotator musculature of the stance leg (see figure 7.31). Execute the front-twist throw described earlier from a single-leg stance. If throwing from the left side, stand on the right foot. The throw begins with the left foot off the ground and forward of the body, with the ball behind the hip. As the throw is executed, the hips rotate, the arms come forward, and the leg moves back. This will eventually become a smooth, coordinated movement.

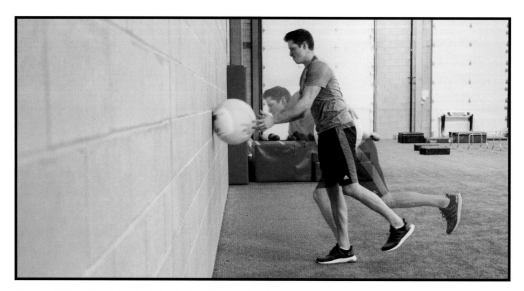

Figure 7.31   Medicine ball single-leg front-twist throw.

Overhead Throws

Overhead throws target the anterior-core musculature and also provide training for the rotator cuff and posterior shoulder. We do not do half-kneeling, tall kneeling, or lunge-position versions. The answer is again found in empiricism and practicality—these versions are not easy to teach or perform. We also do not use the nonbouncing balls for most overhead throws, instead opting for the rubber versions. I do not recommend single-arm throws because the stress of catching with a single arm is too great for the shoulder. Do three sets of 10 reps for overhead throws.

STANDING OVERHEAD THROW
PROGRESSION 1

The standing overhead throw (see figure 7.32) is the starting point for all overhead throwing variations. The drill is similar to a soccer throw-in, but with the feet shoulder-width apart and not staggered. Use the trunk more than the arms to throw the ball. This is an excellent drill for any throwing athlete. Stand far enough away from the wall so the ball returns on one bounce. Do not catch the ball.

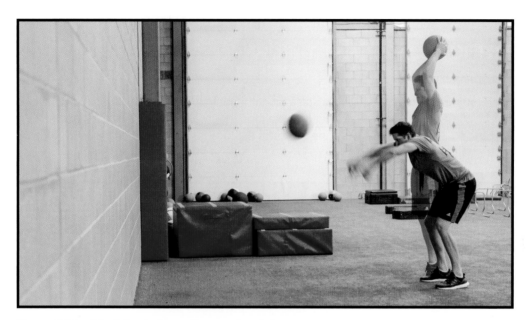

Figure 7.32   Medicine ball standing overhead throw.

STANDING OVERHEAD THROW WITH STAGGERED FEET
PROGRESSION 2

The next progression of the standing overhead throw moves to a staggered stance. This makes the exercise more sport specific and provides greater leg involvement, increased velocity, and a greater diagonal core load. Do not progress to the staggered standing overhead throw until the skill of throwing with the torso has been mastered.

Do three sets of 10 with the right foot in front and then three sets of 10 with the left foot in front.

STANDING OVERHEAD THROW WITH STEP
PROGRESSION 3

This throw is the same as the standing overhead throw in a staggered stance, except instead of a static, staggered stance you are now stepping into the throw. Again, the velocity increases, as does the stress on the posterior shoulder. Stepping and throwing now has more similarity to any overhead throwing or striking sport.

Chest Throws

Chest throws are not really a core exercise but are included with our medicine ball work. They develop the power of the pushing and pressing muscles. The key to chest throws is that they take the strength developed in exercises such as the bench press and create a transfer to many contact sports skills that involve pushing an opponent. Chest throws are basically our upper body plyometric exercise. Please note we do not use exercises such as plyometric push-ups because they have been shown to be hard on the shoulders and the wrists.

▶ TALL KNEELING CHEST THROW
PROGRESSION 1

The first chest throw progression starts in tall kneeling (see figure 7.33). This exercise can be done from a strict tall kneeling position to emphasize upper body power, but we tend to let the athletes drop the hips and explode through to teach linking the hips to the hands. Do three sets of 10 throws.

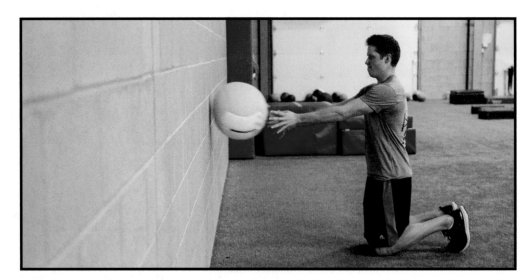

Figure 7.33   Medicine ball tall kneeling chest throw.

STANDING CHEST THROW
PROGRESSION 2

Progression 2 moves to standing in a parallel stance. Here we encourage the athlete to use the hips and explode. Athletes begin in an athletic stance, with the feet slightly wider than the shoulders and the hips and knees slightly flexed. Do three sets of 10 throws.

STEPPING CHEST THROWS
PROGRESSION 3

Progression 3 begins in a staggered stance with the right foot back. The athlete drives off the left foot and steps toward the wall. Do five reps on each side.

SINGLE-ARM ROTATIONAL CHEST THROW
PROGRESSION 4

Progression 4 combines a rotational throw with a chest throw. The chest throw is done with one arm from the same staggered stance used previously. The emphasis is on adding a trunk rotation component to a unilateral upper body throw.

Do three sets of 10 reps with each arm.

FOOTBALL-SPECIFIC STANCE WORK
PROGRESSION 5

For football players, we do throws from a three-point and a low two-point stance depending on position. Defensive linemen begin in a three-point stance and throw from both left and right stances moving toward the wall, linking hips and hands.

Offensive linemen do the previous version as well as a drop-step version that mimics pass protection.

Note: Generally we group our power exercises together and alternate sets of throws with sets of lower body plyometrics. This allows for a preworkout "power period" that addresses lower body power, upper body power, and core power. Pairing jumps and throws allows greater rest than would otherwise be provided if these exercises were done alone.

Core training may be the area of functional training that has changed most significantly. A well-designed core program can have a positive influence on health and all areas of performance. Design your core program to include antirotation exercises, antilateral flexion exercises, diagonal patterns, and medicine ball throws. The core program must be well rounded and well designed to hit all the key areas.

CASE STUDY: REGAINING HEALTH AND VELOCITY

Craig Breslow, a Red Sox pitcher and Yale grad, is known as the smartest man in baseball. Craig trained at Mike Boyle Strength and Conditioning in preparation for the 2015 Major League Baseball season. Breslow's goal was to rebound after a difficult year dealing with shoulder issues. A big part of Craig's training involved medicine ball work to develop the total-body power so important to successful pitching. He did medicine ball training in every session, working through all the progressions to gain power production from the ground to his hands. The result was a healthy spring with an ERA of 0.00 and an increase in velocity.

REFERENCES

Boyle, K.L, J. Olinick, and C. Lewis. 2010. The value of blowing up a balloon. *North American Journal of Sports Physical Therapy.* 5 (3): 179-188.

Cook, G. 1997. Functional Training for the Torso. *Strength and Conditioning.* 19 (2): 14-19.

Cook, G., and B. Jones. *Kettlebells From the Ground Up* (DVD). Functional Movement Systems.

Porterfield, J., and C. DeRosa. 1998. *Mechanical Low Back Pain.* Philadelphia: Saunders.

Sahrmann, S. 2002. *Diagnosis and Treatment of Movement Impairment Syndromes.* St. Louis: Mosby.

Upper Body Training

Many books and articles detail how to do upper body strength exercises. Unfortunately, in spite of all the advice to the contrary, athletes still overemphasize the development of the "mirror muscles" in the chest and arms that contribute to a muscular appearance. This chapter reinforces the need for a balance between pressing and pulling and to emphasize the use of chin-ups, rows, and variations to prevent shoulder injury.

Functional upper body exercise can be divided primarily into pushing and pulling. Other single-joint movements may not be truly functional and work muscles only in isolation. Although single-joint movements may be necessary in corrective or stabilization exercises, the key to functional upper body training is the balance between pushing and pulling.

PULLING FOR INJURY PREVENTION

Most strength training programs place little emphasis on pulling movements such as chin-ups and rows. Although many articles written over the last 50 years have cited pull-ups and chin-ups as keys to upper back development, most athletes ignore these exercises for one simple reason: Pull-ups and chin-ups are just too hard. These athletes instead perform lat pull-downs for the muscles of the upper back under the mistaken assumption that this is all that is necessary, and many completely ignore rowing movements. This type of unbalanced programming often leads to overdevelopment of the pressing muscles, postural problems, and shoulder injury.

An essential goal of a sound upper body program is to equally emphasize all the major upper body movement patterns. Unfortunately, few athletes value the development of back musculature. They'd rather work on building up their chests, a preference that reflects the limits of their (and perhaps their trainers') muscle magazine education.

A well-designed upper body program should include a proportional number of sets of horizontal pulling (rowing), vertical pulling (chin-up), overhead pressing, and supine pressing exercises. In simple terms, there should be a set of pulling exercise for every set of pushing exercise. In the vast majority of strength programs, this is not the case. Most conventional programs generally offer lots of pressing and very little pulling.

Table 8.1   Determining a 1 Repetition Max

100.00%	95.00%	92.50%	90.00%	87.50%	85.00%	82.50%	80.00%	77.50%	75.00%	72.50%	70.00%
1RM	2RM	3RM	4RM	5RM	6RM	7RM	8RM	9RM	10RM	11RM	12RM
120	114	111	108	105	102	99	96	93	90	87	84
125	119	116	113	109	106	103	100	97	94	91	88
130	124	120	117	114	111	107	104	101	98	94	91
135	128	125	122	118	115	111	108	105	101	98	95
140	133	130	126	123	119	116	112	109	105	102	98
145	138	134	131	127	123	120	116	112	109	105	102
150	143	139	135	131	128	124	120	116	113	109	105
155	147	143	140	136	132	128	124	120	116	112	109
160	152	148	144	140	136	132	128	124	120	116	112
165	157	153	149	144	140	136	132	128	124	120	116
170	162	157	153	149	145	140	136	132	128	123	119
175	166	162	158	153	149	144	140	136	131	127	123
180	171	167	162	158	153	149	144	140	135	131	126
185	176	171	167	162	157	153	148	143	139	134	130
190	181	176	171	166	162	157	152	147	143	138	133
195	185	180	176	171	166	161	156	151	146	141	137
200	190	185	180	175	170	165	160	155	150	145	140
205	195	190	185	179	174	169	164	159	154	149	144
210	200	194	189	184	179	173	168	163	158	152	147
215	204	199	194	188	183	177	172	167	161	156	151
220	209	204	198	193	187	182	176	171	165	160	154
225	214	208	203	197	191	186	180	174	169	163	158
230	219	213	207	201	196	190	184	178	173	167	161

This overemphasis on pushing and pressing can lead to postural problems because of the overdevelopment of the pectorals and underdevelopment of the scapular (shoulder blade) retractors. More important, a program that does not provide an equal number of pulling and pushing movements predisposes athletes to overuse shoulder injuries, especially rotator cuff issues.

The incidence of rotator cuff problems among athletes who prioritize bench-pressing is extremely high. In my opinion, this is due less to the bench press itself and more to the lack of an equivalent number of pulling exercises.

The ratio of pulling to pushing strength is best estimated by comparing an athlete's maximum chin-up to her maximum bench-press weight. Consideration must be given to body weight, but athletes capable of bench-pressing well over their body weight should also be capable of pulling their body weight plus additional external load, regardless of their size. In fact, we estimate a 1 RM chin-up by adding chin-up max to body weight. The total number should be equal to or greater than the bench press. For example, if a 200-pound athlete can do 45 pounds in the chin-up for five repetitions, his 1RM would be 280 based on table 8.1. To use the chart for chin-ups determine the total weight used (in this case 245 lbs). Then find 245 in the 5 RM column. Slide over to the left to see the 1 RM in the 1 RM column. If the athlete could bench-press significantly more than 280, he would be considered at risk of injury from a lack of push–pull balance.

100.00%	95.00%	92.50%	90.00%	87.50%	85.00%	82.50%	80.00%	77.50%	75.00%	72.50%	70.00%
1RM	2RM	3RM	4RM	5RM	6RM	7RM	8RM	9RM	10RM	11RM	12RM
235	223	217	212	206	200	194	188	182	176	170	165
240	228	222	216	210	204	198	192	186	180	174	168
245	233	227	221	214	208	202	196	190	184	178	172
250	238	231	225	219	213	206	200	194	188	181	175
255	242	236	230	223	217	210	204	198	191	185	179
260	247	241	234	228	221	215	208	202	195	189	182
265	252	245	239	232	225	219	212	205	199	192	186
270	257	250	243	236	230	223	216	209	203	196	189
275	261	254	248	241	234	227	220	213	206	199	193
280	266	259	252	245	238	231	224	217	210	203	196
285	271	264	257	249	242	235	228	221	214	207	200
290	276	268	261	254	247	239	232	225	218	210	203
295	280	273	266	258	251	243	236	229	221	214	207
300	285	278	270	263	255	248	240	233	225	218	210
305	290	282	275	267	259	252	244	236	229	221	214
310	295	287	279	271	264	256	248	240	233	225	217
315	299	291	284	276	268	260	252	244	236	228	221
320	304	296	288	280	272	264	256	248	240	232	224
325	309	301	293	284	276	268	260	252	244	236	228
330	314	305	297	289	281	272	264	256	248	239	231
335	318	310	302	293	285	276	268	260	251	243	235
340	323	315	306	298	289	281	272	264	255	247	238
345	328	319	311	302	293	285	276	267	259	250	242
350	333	324	315	306	298	289	280	271	263	254	245

Take a moment to quickly figure out your push–pull ratio. Find your chin-up plus body-weight RM and then simply slide over to the far left for a 1RM number. Next, do the same for the bench press. Remember that the chin-up is body weight plus weight on the belt, while the bench press is just weight on the bar.

A properly designed strength program for an athlete should include at least three sets of a chin-up variation per week as well as a minimum of three sets of two rowing movements per week. See table 8.2.

Table 8.2   Chin-Ups of Selected Groups (Elbows to Full Extension)

Elite male (National Hockey League)	45×10
NFL lineman (320 pounds; 145 kg)	BW×7+
NFL skill position	45×10
College male (Division 1)	45×5-10
Elite female (Olympic gold medalist, 152 pounds; 69 kg)	25×10
College female (Division 1)	BW×10

These numbers are not averages but examples from top performers. They are provided merely to indicate what is possible in a program with proper design and proper emphasis.

An important principle in program design is to use numerous variations of the same type of movement. Either the specific type of vertical and horizontal pull should change every three weeks or the number of repetitions should change every three weeks; in some cases, both should change.

STRENGTH STANDARDS

I love the idea of standards. Dan John's strength standard is simple:

Bench = front squat = clean
We no longer front squat, so we can amend this to:

Bench = split squat = clean = chin-up

Many readers will take offense to this, but if you train athletes this could not be more true. The reality is that if an athlete can bench-press 300 pounds (136 kg), he can also split-squat 120-pound (55 kg) dumbbells for eight repetitions and clean 265 pounds (120 kg) five times (based on table 8.1, all projected to a 300-pound max). If he can't the reason is simple: He isn't trying hard enough.

Dan provides a standard for high school football as follows:

Clean: 205 pounds (93 kg)

Bench: 205 pounds (93 kg)

Squat: 255 pounds (116 kg)

Clean + jerk: 165 pounds (75 kg)

Not really impressive numbers, but they add up to a good athlete who has spent some time in the weight room doing the right things.

Here's another way to look at standards:

Bench 5RM = hang clean 5RM = rear-foot-elevated split squat 5RM = chin-up 5RM

The chin-up 5RM can come from table 8.1 but still needs to be equal to the bench press 5RM.

If my athletes can do this I know they are working hard in all areas. If they can exceed their bench 5RM in the hang clean and rear-foot-elevated spit squat, all the better. I always tell my athletes, "If you are going to stink at one lift, stink at the bench. It's the least important."

These standards apply to women also. A female who can bench 135 pounds (61 kg) will most often far exceed the chin-up standard but should also be able to hang-clean 135 pounds and do split squats with 55-pound (25 kg) dumbbells for eight repetitions (that's 110 pounds in table 8.1; 110 × 8 = 135 1RM).

VERTICAL PULLING MOVEMENTS

Variation is the key to continued strength gain. It is important to vary either the type of exercise or the loading pattern every three weeks.

CHIN-UP
PROGRESSION 1A

The chin-up is the easiest of the body-weight vertical pulling movements because of the supinated grip (palms facing in toward the body) and corresponding gain in biceps assistance. Use a 12- to 14-inch (30 to 36 cm) grip width. Essential techniques for all the vertical pulling movements are to fully extend the elbows and to allow the scapulae to elevate slightly. Athletes should not be allowed to cheat. A kipping pull-up is cheating, and don't let anyone tell you otherwise. The only thing kipping is good for is ego inflation.

Over the first eight weeks, don't be concerned about variety. Beginners need less variety than advanced trainees.

Chin-ups and the variations are best cycled in the strength program to correspond with the other major exercises (hang clean, split squat, bench press). Do three sets of 8 to 10 chin-ups, three to five sets of 5, and three to five sets of 3.

Although machines are available to assist with chin-ups and pull-ups, you can set up a much simpler system for far less money. Simply loop a heavy-duty resistance band (such as the ones made by Perform Better, which are well constructed and come in heavy, medium, and light resistances) over the pull-up bar.

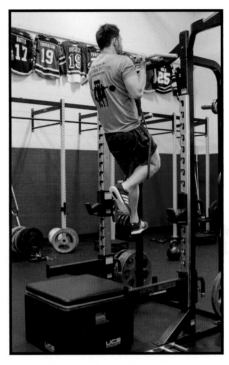

Figure 8.1   Assisted chin-up.

The athlete places one knee in the band and lowers to the start position. The elastic energy of the band assists in the ascent. The athlete can work down progressively from heavy to light resistance bands and then to unassisted full body weight. Larger or weaker athletes can also stand with the foot in the band to better benefit from the elastic energy. An athlete can also stand on a band placed across the rack on the J hooks used to bench press. I prefer standing on the band (see figure 8.1), but the setup for more than one athlete can be difficult.

Eight-Week Chin-Up Progression

This program is intended to be done two times per week only. Once an athlete can perform one unassisted chin-up, she can use the eight-week program in table 8.3. It is not unusual for athletes to advance from one chin-up to five after this eight-week progression.

Athletes who can perform more than 10 chin-ups should use a dip belt to add additional weight. We have moved away from the higher-rep chin-up tests and developed a system where the athletes are pushed to get strong. If an athlete can do 10 chin-ups or pull-ups, the next test is with a dip belt at 25 pounds (11 kg).

Using the dip belt lets an athlete cycle the vertical pulling movements while doing the other major lifts. When the program calls for three repetitions, increase the weight and perform sets of three repetitions. It is not unusual for our male athletes to use 90 pounds (41 kg) or more for sets of three and for our female athletes to use 25 to 45 pounds (11 to 20 kg).

A healthy athlete who can perform five assisted chin-ups with a heavy band should never do pull-downs. Extremely overweight athletes who have a poor ratio of strength to body weight should perform pull-downs. Young kids and older adults may also benefit from pull-downs. However, there is no rationale for pull-downs by healthy athletes who are capable of chin-ups or assisted chin-ups. Pull-downs are simply an easy way out for people who do not want to do chin-ups.

Table 8.3   Eight-Week Unassisted Chin-Up Program

Week 1	4 × 1 (This means four single repetitions, with a 3- to 5-second eccentric contraction at the end of the last rep.)
Week 2	1 × 2, 3 × 1
Week 3	2 × 2, 2 × 1
Week 4	3 × 2, 1 × 1
Week 5	4 × 2
Week 6	1 × 3, 3 × 2
Week 7	2 × 3, 2 × 2
Week 8	3 × 3, 1 × 2

PARALLEL-GRIP PULL-UP
PROGRESSION 1B

This excellent upper body pulling exercise is similar to the chin-up but targets the forearm and elbow flexors (brachialis and brachioradialis) because of the neutral hand position. Parallel-grip pull-ups can be done on a pull-up bar equipped with a V handle or parallel handles (see figure 8.2). Execution is the same as for the chin-up; only the hand position differs. The parallel-grip pull-up is similar in difficulty to the chin-up because of the increased forearm flexor contribution. Athletes with shoulder or wrist issues may find the parallel-grip version more comfortable than either chin-ups or pull-ups.

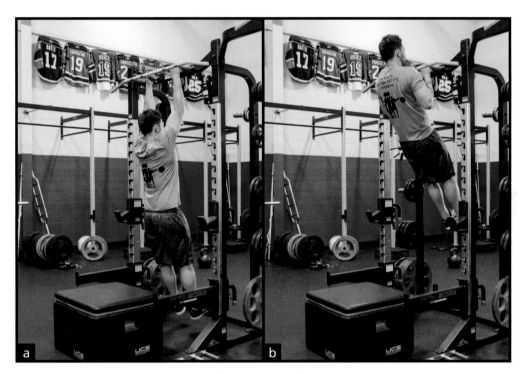

Figure 8.2   Parallel-grip pull-up.

PULL-UP
PROGRESSION 2

The pull-up is a more difficult exercise than the chin-up or parallel-grip pull-up. In the pull-up the hands are pronated (palms forward). There is less assistance from the muscles of the upper arm and correspondingly more stress on the back muscles, which significantly increases the difficulty. The pull-up should be the third exercise done in the upper-body program, after a minimum of three weeks of chin-ups and parallel-grip pull-ups. The pull-up is also the least shoulder-friendly version because of the abducted and externally rotated position of the shoulder. Avoid these with any athletes with shoulder issues.

STERNUM CHIN-UP
PROGRESSION 3

The sternum chin-up is a difficult variation for even advanced athletes. To do the sternum chin-up, pull the sternum up to the bar rather than pull the chin above the bar (see figure 8.3). This requires using the scapular retractors to a greater degree and increases the range of motion by three to four inches (8 to 10 cm).

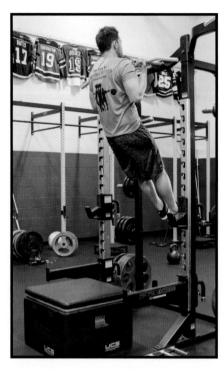

Figure 8.3   Sternum chin-up.

PULL-DOWN VARIATIONS
REGRESSION 1

I never thought I'd be including lat pull-downs in this book. I have always advocated for chin-ups and pull-ups as superior choices. But, as always, times change. If you asked me today what to do for upper body pulling I might tell you to do body-weight rows on the TRX or rings (featured in the next section on horizontal pulling) and then follow that up with one of the variations of the pull-down you are about to read about, especially if you had any shoulder issues.

Think of the suspension rows as the heavy horizontal pulling exercise and the lat pull-downs as the lighter vertical pull. As a matter of fact, from here on in, I'll just call them *pull-downs* because pull-down exercises work a lot more than just the lats. They work the lats, the lower and middle trapezius, the rhomboids, and the serratus, to name a few muscles. And, by the way, please do not ever call them lateral pull-downs. *Lat* is short for *latissimus* (as in latissimus dorsi) not *lateral*.

Why the change of heart? Some people (primarily younger athletes and female athletes) are simply not able to do vertical pulls such as chin-ups and pull-ups well. As much as I like them for elite athletes, I have been guilty of occasionally jamming a square peg into a round hole. In addition, older clients or those with shoulder issues have trouble with body-weight vertical pulls such as pull-ups but usually have zero issues with heavy horizontal pulls. The reality is that a suspension exercise such as the TRX or ring row is far more scalable than the pull-up. I know, we can use bands, we can do isometrics, we can do eccentrics, but not everyone can do these things well. We might have to accept the idea that for some people pull-downs may present an acceptable alternative.

What we see in our facility are people overusing their upper traps and biceps in vertical pulling exercises such as chin-ups and pull-ups. I don't see this nearly as much in the suspension rows. The TRX and ring row are fully scalable exercises that you can progress or regress easily, something far more difficult to do well with a pull-up or chin-up.

Another reason I like pull-downs again is the invention of the functional trainer. No, not the person standing on the BOSU, the machine with the two arms.

Think about this. Why did we used to do all our pull-downs with both hands on a fixed bar? Because everyone else did and we really had no other choice. For years the pull-down bar or the V-handle or whatever handle you chose to use determined how the shoulder would function in the pull-down exercise. Suddenly companies such as FreeMotion and Keiser developed units they called functional trainers with two independent arms and two independent handles. In the process, a whole new group of shoulder-friendly exercises was born. We could now select the best hand position instead of having the hand position selected for us, and we could use both arms at the same time but separately. The functional trainer became like a dumbbell for the shoulder in pulling patterns.

Why does this matter? Well, how many athletes do you know with shoulder problems? Lots, right? Do you know that one of the primary causes of shoulder problems is the constant rubbing of the rotator cuff tendons under the acromial arch? The rubbing leads to attrition of the rotator cuff tendon, much like pulling a rope back and forth across a rock. If you pull with a fixed bar, you rub the same portion of the tendon under the acromion every time.

Now grab the handles of a functional trainer. What's funny is that most people try to mimic the position of the straight bar. This is just dumb. Our instructions are clear: Start thumb down (internally rotated at the shoulder). Finish thumb up (externally rotated at the shoulder). If I move from a thumb-down position to a thumb-up position, what action have I added to my pull-down? External rotation! I have made the shoulder move in a very joint-friendly, spiral, diagonal pattern, and I've added a little rotator cuff twist. This exercise just went from zero to hero in my book.

Another big teaching point comes courtesy of my friend Michol Dalcourt. Tell your clients to push the chest toward the machine. Guess what? You just got them to retract their scapulae just like you wanted them to, but you didn't need to cue them to pinch the shoulder blades. Dalcourt made a great point years ago in a seminar: You can't push your chest forward and shrug your shoulders at the same time. Pushing the chest forward is retraction. Shrugging is elevation. Want to eliminate shrugging at the top of the pull-down? Cue chest to bar, not bar to chest. There are no muscles that move the chest forward, only muscles that move the shoulders back. However, the result of the two cues (shoulders back versus chest forward) can be totally different. Try it. It works every time.

X PULL-DOWN
BASELINE

We use the term *X pull-down* because the arms begin crossed (see figure 8.4). With the independent handles of the functional trainer, you can now adduct and depress the scapulae, extend the shoulders, and incorporate some external rotation. This adds a frontal- and transverse-plane component to what was basically a sagittal exercise.

Note: If you don't have a functional trainer but want the benefits, simply do your pull-downs one arm at a time off a cable column. Also, if you get above body weight on the pull-down machine, it might be time for chin-ups.

As mentioned already, start with the arms crossed and the thumbs down.

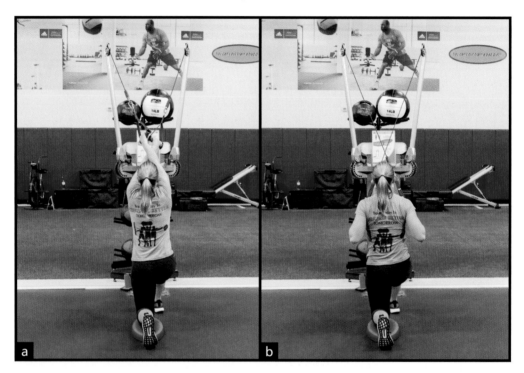

Figure 8.4   X pull-down.

ALTERNATING X PULL-DOWN
PROGRESSION 1

Want to add a scapular stability component? Holding one arm in the down position results in more low trap and rhomboid work (think W from the Y-T-W series presented later in the chapter), while the opposite side gets retraction, depression, extension, horizontal adduction, and external rotation. Talk about bang for the buck. Alternating X pull-downs combines a scapular stability exercise with a vertical pulling exercise.

Want a little variety? Try alternating without the crossed grip. These three variations provide a selection of shoulder-friendly exercises for all our athletes and clients.

Does this mean we no longer do any pull-ups or chin-ups? No. What it does mean is that we match the right exercise with the right athlete. If we have young athletes capable of doing pull-ups and chin-ups, you can bet they will do them. If we have older clients with neck and cervical issues or younger clients with strength issues, you'll see the suspension row, pull-down combination.

HORIZONTAL PULLING MOVEMENTS

Horizontal pulling movements, or rowing movements, are extremely important and must be included and prioritized in the upper body program. Rows are a priority because they are the true antagonistic movement to the bench press. Although chin-ups and their variations are important, rowing movements target both the muscles and the movement patterns that directly oppose those trained (and often overtrained) with the bench press. Despite their importance, rows are frequently omitted from strength programs or are performed with limited intent.

Rowing motions in functional training are undergoing great change. Recent advances in athletic training and physical therapy have illustrated that the body is linked posteriorly in a diagonal pattern. Force is transmitted from the ground through the leg to the hip and then across the SI joint (sacroiliac joint) into the opposite latissimus dorsi (the lat, a surface back muscle) and shoulder complex. The keys in this system of cross-linkage are the gluteus medius and quadratus lumborum, which stabilize the pelvis, and the hip rotator group, which stabilizes the hip.

The hip rotator group is of particular importance because all force originating at the ground, whether a golf swing or a home run, must be transferred through a strong, flexible, and stable hip to properly transfer to the upper body. Until very recently, this vital group has been effectively ignored. The hip rotators are the rotator cuff of the lower body but do not get the respect and attention that the rotator cuff muscles in the shoulder get. The hip rotators must be given particular attention in program design. Rowing movements done with a cable column can help strengthen this undertrained area.

DUMBBELL ROW
PROGRESSION 1

The dumbbell row is the simplest of rowing movements and can help beginners learn proper back position, a skill that can transfer to a number of lifts. In spite of being a relatively simple movement, the dumbbell row may be one of the most difficult exercises to teach.

Begin in a wide squat-type stance, with the knees out over the feet. Lean forward and place one hand on a bench to stabilize the torso and take stress off the low back. The back stays slightly arched, and the abdominals are tight. Concentrate first on moving the scapula and then the elbow to bring the dumbbell back to the hip (see figure 8.5). This movement is great for beginners but does not work the hip rotator group because of the double-leg stance. Do three sets of 5 to 10 repetitions, depending on the training phase.

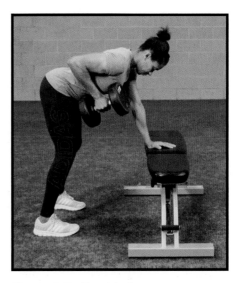

Figure 8.5   Dumbbell row.

▶ CAT–COW
REGRESSION 1

We have developed a few regressions to help teach the dumbbell row. One of the major failures of the dumbbell row is the inability to maintain a slight arch in the back. Cat–cow (see figure 8.6) is a yoga exercise designed to teach athletes to move the spine into flexion and extension. We use it as an awareness drill to teach an athlete to keep a slight arch in the back during the row. The athlete starts on all fours and alternately

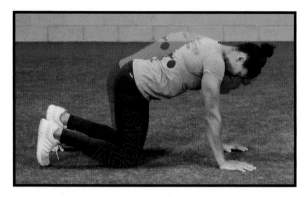

Figure 8.6   Cat–cow.

creates a hump like an angry cat and then reverses to a substantial arch. Teaching spinal movement without hip movement reinforces the start position for the dumbbell row. One or two sets of two or three repetitions is often enough to create the awareness needed.

BENCH STRADDLE ROW
REGRESSION 2

Another flaw in the dumbbell row is the inability to keep the knees wide in a squat stance. Having an athlete straddle a bench can reinforce the knees-out position. If the row is being performed with the right hand, the athlete stands parallel to the bench with the left hand on the bench and the left leg on the opposite side, the inside of the knee lightly touching the bench (see figure 8.7). In this position, the left knee is unable to cave in, and a better body position is maintained. The combination of a few cat–cow repetitions and a straddle position is often all that is needed to clean up dumbbell row technique.

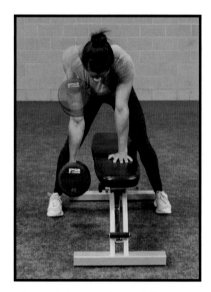

Figure 8.7   Bench straddle row.

SUSPENSION TRAINER INVERTED ROW
PROGRESSION 2

The suspension trainer inverted row may be the best exercise not done on a regular basis. Inverted rows are a wonderfully simple yet challenging movement that teaches torso stabilization and develops strength in the scapular retractors and rear deltoid. Although the movement appears simple, the inverted row is often a humbling exercise for even the strongest athletes. Athletes with strong pressing muscles are often unpleasantly surprised at how few quality inverted rows they can perform.

The advent of suspension trainers such as the TRX or rings has made the inverted row simple to do in any facility that has power racks or wall mounts. The ability to lengthen or shorten the

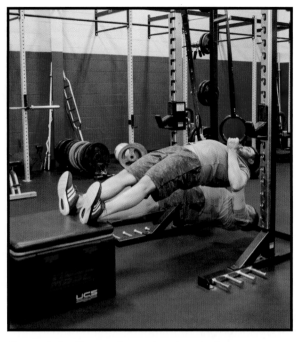

Figure 8.8   Suspension trainer inverted row.

straps has made it easy to scale the exercise to any athlete at any strength level. In the first edition of this book, the inverted row was a humbling exercise that wasn't always a great programming fit based on equipment setup. The suspension straps have changed all that. We no longer recommend the bar version of the exercise and use only the TRX or ring version. In addition to the ease of adapting the rings or TRX to any strength level, the suspension trainers also allow the shoulders to move from internal rotation to external rotation by beginning in a thumb-down position and ending in a thumb-up position. This benefit is huge for shoulder health.

To perform the inverted row, set up the suspension trainer with the handles at approximately waist height. The key is to figure out the body angle that will be the best challenge. Because of the adjustability of the suspension trainers, the body can be positioned at any angle. Maximum difficulty is obtained with the body parallel to the floor and the feet on a bench placed approximately three-quarters of a body length away. With the feet on the bench and the hands on the handles the torso is perfectly straight. The toes are pointed up, and the feet are together. From this position, simply pull the chest to the handles (see figure 8.8). Most athletes are unable to touch the chest to the handles after the first few repetitions because of weakness in the scapular retractors and posterior deltoid. This exercise stresses not only the upper back but also the entire torso. To increase the functional overload of the torso muscles, advanced athletes can perform this exercise with the addition of a weight vest.

Do three sets of 8 to 10 repetitions, and attempt to decrease the angle (as measured from the floor) every week until the feet are on the bench.

SINGLE-ARM, SINGLE-LEG ROW (STATIC HIPS)

BASELINE

The single-arm, single-leg row is the first exercise in the rowing progression to address the hip rotators as stabilizers. It requires an adjustable cable column set at approximately waist height. To do this exercise, stand on one foot to execute a row with the opposite hand (see figure 8.9).

The single-leg stance elevates the row to a complex exercise that develops proprioception, strength, and stability in the ankle, knee, and hip. The single-arm, single-leg row should initially emphasize stabilization. Attempt to stabilize the ankle, knee, and hip while rowing to a position on the rib cage just below the chest. As in all cable rowing movements, shoulder rotator cuff work can be added by beginning with the

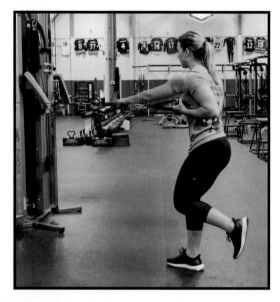

Figure 8.9   Single-arm, single-leg row.

thumb down and finishing with the thumb up. The rotator cuff becomes involved in the row as the shoulder position changes.

Do three sets of 5 to 10 repetitions, depending on the training phase.

SINGLE-ARM, SINGLE-LEG ROW (DYNAMIC HIPS)

PROGRESSION 1

The only difference between the dynamic and static versions of this exercise is that the athlete is allowed to reach into the cable column in the dynamic version. The reach involves trunk rotation and hip internal rotation, and a load is placed on the lateral (external) hip rotators as the rowing movement is completed. This movement dynamically stresses the body from ankle to shoulder. In a sense, the athlete is allowed to "cheat" by increasing hip movement. Do three sets of 5 to 10 repetitions, depending on the training phase.

▶ SINGLE-ARM, DOUBLE-LEG ROTATIONAL ROW

PROGRESSION 2

The single-arm, double-leg rotational row is borrowed from performance enhancement expert Mark Verstegen's EXOS team. It is an extremely dynamic movement that incorporates leg extension, hip internal rotation, and trunk rotation into a total-body rowing exercise.

This functional and integrated exercise is best described as half squat, half row. I believe this relatively new exercise will soon be a staple in all functional training programs. The best part about the single-arm, double-leg rotational row is the way it mimics the mechanics of direction change.

To teach the exercise I often tell our athletes to envision the stop-and-start mechanics of a lateral shuffle. Assume a position with the shoulders aligned with the line of pull of a cable column or low pulley. Reach across the body to grasp the handle, and pull the handle to the hip while standing up tall (see figure 8.10).

The squatting muscles are used in conjunction with the rowing muscles to simultaneously extend the legs, rotate the trunk, and extend the shoulder. The only muscles not stressed by this exercise are the pressing muscles. Try to visualize the forces needed to brake and change direction, and the exercise will take on whole new relevance. Do three sets of 5 to 10 repetitions, depending on the training phase.

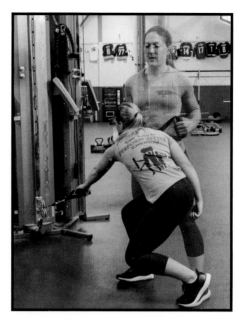

Figure 8.10 Single-arm, double-leg rotational row.

UPPER BODY PRESSING EXERCISES

This section focuses on functional upper body strength rather than the bench press. I want to make it clear that athletes we train perform bench presses, dumbbell bench presses, and numerous other variations of supine pressing movements. I am not against the bench press, but my philosophy is balanced training in which performance in one relatively unimportant lift is not overemphasized. In functional training it is important that the combination of supine and overhead pressing should not take up more than 30 minutes twice per week. Any additional time spent on pressing movements detracts from the training of other muscle groups and disturbs the balance of the program.

Table 8.4 presents a set of general guidelines that are helpful in program design and strength evaluation. The guidelines are provided to help coaches, trainers, and athletes achieve greater balance among the different supine pressing exercises. You can improve your bench press numbers by increasing other related lifts. Often athletes are so focused on one lift that they actually retard their progress. Strive for balanced pressing strength in which strength is developed at a variety of angles (incline, overhead) along with stability (by using dumbbells). One angle or one action should not become dominant. All upper body dumbbell work is prescribed with these guidelines in mind. Beginners need to increase weights slowly to develop the necessary balance and stability to lift heavier weights.

Table 8.4 Proper Strength Relationship in Upper-Body Presses

Bench press (example) 300 lb (136 kg) max	Incline bench press 240 lb (109 kg; 80% of bench max)	Dumbbell bench press 95 × 5 (64% of bench max / 2 to get dumbbell weight)	Dumbbell incline bench press 77 × 5 (80% of dumbbell bench max)

This chart shows the amount of weight an athlete should be able to lift after a proper training program to develop balanced upper body pressing strength.

PUSH-UP
BASELINE

One of the most underrated exercises in the upper body program, push-ups are pressing movements that require no equipment and offer numerous variations. The push-up is an excellent exercise for larger athletes who need to improve their strength-to-body-weight ratios. For this reason alone push-ups are a great exercise in football training programs. Another great advantage of the push-up is that it combines upper body training with core development. Many larger athletes or athletes who are weak throughout the core have difficulty maintaining the proper body position for a push-up. In addition, push-ups work the shoulder blade area in a way that the bench press cannot.

FEET-ELEVATED PUSH-UP
PROGRESSION 1

The feet-elevated push-up (see figure 8.11) is the simplest way to increase difficulty. Athletes who find the push-up easy can elevate the feet from 12 to 24 inches (30 to 60 cm) to increase the difficulty without adding any external resistance. From here, athletes can progress to the BOSU push-up or add a weighted vest or a plate on the back.

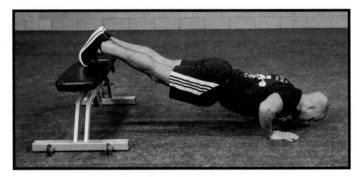

Figure 8.11   Feet-elevated push-up.

BOSU BALL PUSH-UP
PROGRESSION 3

The BOSU ball push-up (see figure 8.12) can be done in a feet-elevated version or with a weight vest. It develops proprioception in the upper body and the torso and places the hands in a much more sports-general position.

Do three sets of 5 to 10 repetitions, depending on the training phase. More push-up repetitions can be done in endurance phases.

The proper progression for push-ups is illustrated in figure 8.13.

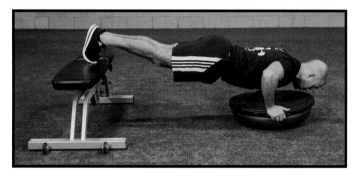

Figure 8.12   BOSU ball push-up.

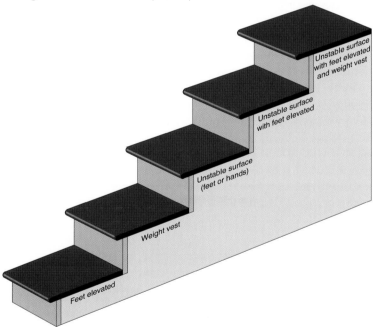

Figure 8.13   Push-up progression.

STANDING CABLE PRESS
REGRESSION 1

Single-arm standing cable presses can be done on any adjustable cable column and might be the most functional way to press. The AT Sports Flex mentioned in the Training Tools section of chapter 4 allows for a great double-arm standing version of this exercise. The exercise can also be done unilaterally. An added benefit of the standing cable press is that the core is loaded in standing.

OVERHEAD PRESSING

Overhead pressing is another area not covered in the first edition of *Functional Training for Sports*. In many ways, the thought processes remain the same as we discussed in the pulling chapter and core chapters. We do not use a straight bar, we choose unilateral versions, and we begin with positions that improve stability.

As mentioned in the section on vertical and horizontal pulling, straight bars determine the bar path and the shoulder motion for the lifter. Like the individual handles on the newer functional trainers or the handles of a suspension trainer, dumbbells allow the shoulder to have more freedom. This is a huge plus over using a straight bar for overhead presses. Overhead work will begin in half kneeling to stabilize the lumbar spine and to force the lifter to use the shoulders.

The most common mistake in overhead pressing is creating a backward lean or a lumbar arch that effectively turns the overhead press into an incline press. The backward lean allows the upper pecs to become active as in an incline press. However, the trade-off is a large stress to the lumbar spine.

HALF-KNEELING ALTERNATING KETTLEBELL PRESS
BASELINE

My choice for where to start overhead work is with a half-kneeling stance and kettlebells. The offset nature of the kettlebell produces a natural external rotation moment at the shoulder, and this seems to recruit the subscapularis (a key shoulder stabilizer). Often athletes or clients who complain of overhead presses being uncomfortable will find the alternating kettlebell version to be completely pain free.

Begin with both kettlebells at shoulder level with the thumbs touching the front deltoids. Elbows are about 45 degrees to the torso. Press up with one kettlebell, driving the shoulder into internal rotation (thumb toward the face) (see figure 8.14). Reverse the motion in the descent and switch to the opposite side. Perform three sets of 5 to 10 repetitions.

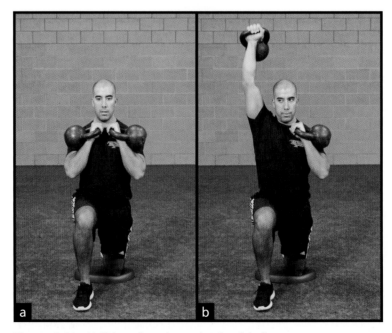

Figure 8.14   Half-kneeling alternating kettlebell press.

BOTTOM-UP KETTLEBELL PRESS
REGRESSION 1

If the half-kneeling alternating press is still painful or uncomfortable, try the bottom-up version. The kettlebell is held bottom up by the handle and pressed as for the previous exercise. The bottom-up position is an even greater recruiter of the shoulder stabilizers and may again surprisingly produce a pain-free overhead press.

HIGH SPLIT ALTERNATING PRESS
PROGRESSION 1

In the high split the lifter moves from the half-kneeling position to a standing position with one foot placed on a 30- to 45-degree incline bench (see figure 8.15). The key is to lean into the front foot to really stabilize the lumbar spine. This is almost a standing version of the half-kneeling position that again forces the lifter to really use the shoulders versus creating a pseudo incline press

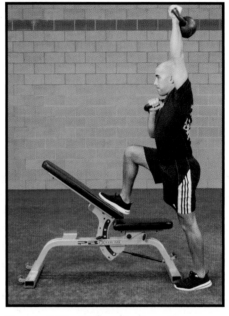

Figure 8.15   High split alternating press.

STANDING ALTERNATING DUMBBELL PRESS
PROGRESSION 2

Once the athlete has learned to press with the shoulders and not arch the back or shift the hips forward to create an incline press, the athlete can move to a more standard standing press position (see figure 8.16). However, dumbbells are still used and alternated from the bottom.

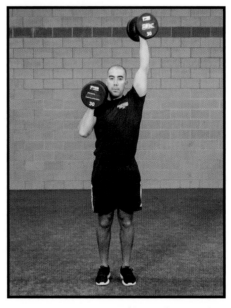

Figure 8.16   Standing alternating dumbbell press.

SCAPULOTHORACIC AND GLENOHUMERAL JOINT TRAINING

Some exercises that initially appear nonfunctional may in fact be useful and improve function at certain joints. The scapulothoracic (shoulder blade–rib cage) joint and glenohumeral (shoulder) joints are two areas that may benefit from isolation exercises to improve their function and at the same time the function of the entire shoulder joint.

The mistake in shoulder training has been to approach it as an either/or proposition. Some coaches operate from the premise that you either believe in functional training or you don't. These coaches view training for the shoulder musculature as multijoint training and tend to avoid any isolation exercises or rotator cuff exercises. The thought process advanced by some of these experts is that any isolation is nonfunctional and a waste of time. I believe that some isolation for both the hip and shoulder joints can be beneficial.

The best approach is to combine overhead presses for strength with exercises to improve shoulder stability for injury prevention. The target of these shoulder prehabilitation exercises should be movement and stabilization of the scapula and the glenohumeral joint.

The function of the scapulothoracic joint and the strength of the rotator cuff are critical for injury reduction. Strengthening the rotator cuff muscles without strengthening the scapular stabilizers does only half the job. Even a strong rotator cuff needs a stable base from which to operate. This stable base is provided by the scapulothoracic joint.

Standing Shoulder Circuit

The standing shoulder circuit uses the AT Sports Flex, which brings scapulothoracic training to an entirely new level in both position and ease of use. The letters Y, T, and W describe the positions in which to perform scapular retraction or movements. The shape of the letter suggests the placement of the arms in relation to the body.

Y = Arms from 45 degrees above shoulder level, with the thumbs pointed up to facilitate external rotation.

T = With the upper arm at a 90-degree angle to the torso and the thumbs pointed up. The key to this position is to retract the scapulae and maintain a 90-degree angle at the shoulder. Many athletes with weak scapular retractors pull the arms down to the sides slightly to substitute action of the lats for that of the scapular retractors. This produces an adduction movement instead of a retraction movement and should be guarded against carefully. The angle should never be less than 90 degrees, which indicates lat substitution.

W = Upper arm at a 45-degree angle to the torso, which emphasizes scapular retraction.

This thought process is simple and probably familiar to many physical therapists and athletic trainers, but the key is in how the athlete thinks about the execution of the movements. The athlete must move the arms by *moving the scapulothoracic joint*, not the reverse. The initial emphasis is on scapulothoracic movement, not glenohumeral movement. This approach changes the exercises from shoulder exercises to scapular stabilizing exercises.

SPORTS FLEX HIGH–LOW (Y–W COMBO)

In the high–low the athlete moves one arm into the W angle and the opposite arm into the Y position (see figure 8.17). I tell my athletes to imagine doing the Gator Chomp at a University of Florida game.

Begin with eight repetitions on one side, and switch to the opposite without resting between exercises.

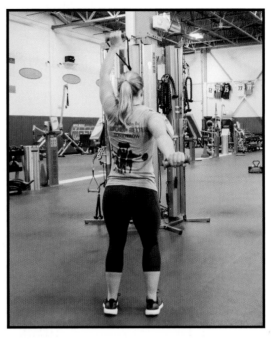

Figure 8.17   Sports Flex high–low (Y–W combo).

SPORTS FLEX T

After doing the Y–W combination, perform eight Ts by adducting the shoulder blades with the arms at 90 degrees (see figure 8.18). In this one we think, *Gimme a T.*

Add 2 repetitions per week, up to sets of 12 repetitions in each position (36 repetitions total). At this point you think about a maintenance program.

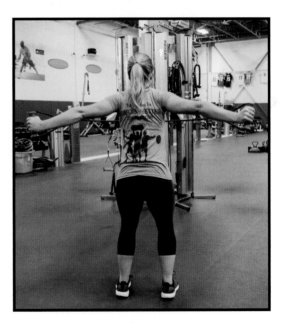

Figure 8.18   Sports Flex T.

STANDING EXTERNAL ROTATION

The first edition did not include any rotator cuff exercises, which may have been a mistake. Although there is still some disagreement about whether or not rotator cuff isolation is needed, we have adopted a "better safe than sorry" approach. Although many so-called experts say isolated rotator cuff work is not necessary, almost every Major League Baseball team still does them. This is a large piece of strong anecdotal evidence.

The best way to perform rotator cuff exercises is in the closed pack position, the point at which the joint surfaces match up ideally (i.e., the ball lines up well in the socket) and the joint is effectively in the best position to work. For the rotator cuff, this is best described as a 90–45 position. For years rotator cuff exercises were done standing or side-lying with the arm at the side and the elbow bent to 90 degrees. This is an extremely nonfunctional position because the muscles never work in that fashion. Instead of 0 degrees of abduction, think of the arm with 90 degrees of abduction but the elbow pointing out at a 45-degree angle (see figure 8.19).

I prefer high repetitions in the 15 to 20 range for rotator cuff work because these muscles are really stabilizers.

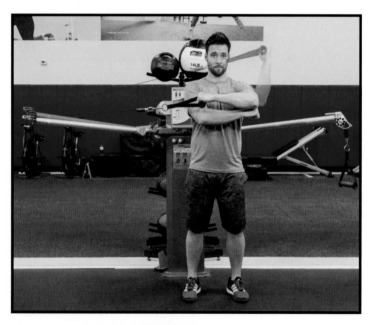

Figure 8.19   Standing external rotation.

CLOSING POINTS ON UPPER BODY TRAINING

The upper body may be the most difficult area to train because of a fascination with training for appearance rather than function. Athletes may be reluctant to perform push-ups instead of bench presses or to work on back muscles they cannot see.

Experimenting with the chin-up and push-up variations can be valuable. Athletes may find that they do not have the torso stability and strength to perform the inverted row or the push-up and thus come to appreciate functional training for the upper body. Don't fight to remove sacred cows such as the bench press; simply incorporate more functional exercises into the program. A slow transition in the upper body area can help overcome resistance to functional training.

Plyometric Training

Training for power may be the most important part of training for an athlete. Ultimately strength should be gained to allow the production of power and speed. Increases in strength that do not produce a concurrent increase in power are really of limited use, particularly in no-collision sports. The truth is that many athletes spend far too much time strength training and far too little time training for power.

The question is not "should we train for power?" but "how do we train for power?" In a perfect world, with a healthy athlete, power training is done in multiple ways. Plyometrics, medicine ball throws (chapter 7), and Olympic lifts (chapter 10) are all effective means by which to develop power output. Each method can be essential in creating a powerful athlete, and all have their place in a well-designed program. The best program uses each of the following three methods.

Method 1: Light-Implement Power Development Light-implement power development is basically medicine ball throwing. Light implements (usually under 5 kilograms) are used to develop power in a number of patterns. The key is that the weight of the implement can be chosen based on the athlete's or client's strengths or needs.

Light-implement power development is generally divided into overhead throws, chest throws, slams, and rotational patterns. For overhead work we rarely exceed 6 pounds (3 kg). For chest throws we use 8- to 10-pound (4 to 5 kg) nonbouncing medicine balls. We generally use the same 8- to 10-pound balls for rotational power. The nonbouncing balls are great because they force the thrower to emphasize the concentric part of the throw.

In this method, light implements are thrown at high velocity. The load is released from the hands. With medicine balls we can more easily access the velocity end of the force velocity curve because the load is light and easy to accelerate. Light implements such as the medicine ball can also be used for lower body power although we rarely do it at MBSC.

Method 2: Body-Weight Power Development   Body-weight power development is basically lower body plyometrics, the subject of the remainder of this chapter. Body-weight power training involves a wide continuum, from a mature, highly elastic professional athlete to a young athlete just learning to jump. Coaches and trainers must be far more careful in plyometric training than with medicine ball training. In medicine ball training the load can be selected and controlled. In plyometric training body weight presents a difficult, but not impossible, constant that must be accounted for.

Unfortunately, body weight is a constant force that can be greatly magnified by gravity. Body-weight power work will develop the power production of the hips and legs, but proper progressions and regressions are essential.

It is important to note that what constitutes warm-up in an athlete's program might be considered body-weight power work for an adult client. Body-weight power plyometric exercises must be prescribed with great care.

Machines such as the Shuttle MVP and Total Gym Jump Trainer (see figure 9.1) are excellent tools for developing power in adult or larger clients such as football linemen and basketball centers and forwards. The Shuttle MVP and Total Gym allow for working at gradually increasing percentages of body weight. A Pilates Reformer or Total Gym can also be used for these purposes. The keys are again the speed component and the eccentric response to gravity.

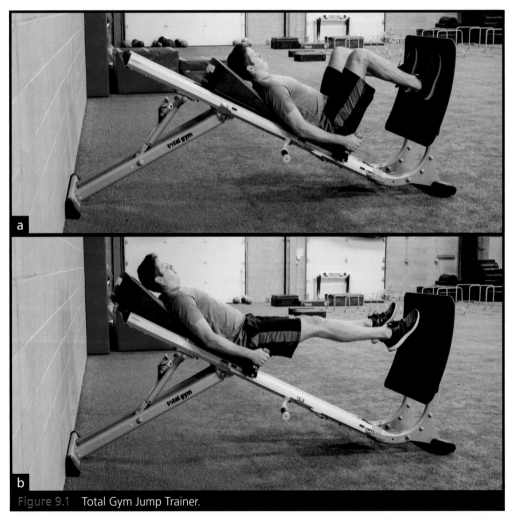

Figure 9.1   Total Gym Jump Trainer.

Method 3: Heavy-Implement Power Development In heavy-implement power work, athletes or clients use heavier external loads in the form of kettlebells or Olympic bars. The vast majority of our clients use this third method. The exclusion might be some of our older athletes or those athletes with chronic back pain. In general, older, noncompetitive clients do not perform Olympic lifts. I think Olympic lifting for adults is a poor choice on the risk–reward or risk–benefit scale. Our healthy adult clients use kettlebell swings for external-load power development. There is a much smaller learning curve and lower loads with the kettlebell.

The big takeaway is that power development is essential for both athletes and nonathletes. Athletes obviously need power work to improve performance, while adults need power work to offset the aging-related loss of fast-twitch capability. A case could be made for adults having greater needs for power work because science has shown that adults lose power faster than strength. However, the process must proceed logically. As we so often mention, the key is to choose the right tool for the right job. As coaches, we often force square pegs into round holes in our desire to use a lift, a tool, or an exercise. What is good for a 20-year-old athlete may be a potential disaster for a young or overweight athlete.

KEY FACTORS IN PLYOMETRIC TRAINING

A coach's likes, dislikes, and areas of expertise should in some ways determine the method used. Coaches who are not comfortable teaching Olympic lifting should refrain from using this skill. However, every athlete should jump and throw medicine balls. These are simple exercises that can be mastered by any coach and any athlete.

At our training facility healthy athletes are exposed daily to all three methods. A combination of Olympic lifts, medicine ball throws, and plyometrics is the best way to develop explosive power, and this can be accomplished safely if certain guidelines are followed. This chapter discusses plyometric training, or using body weight for power development.

One initial point is that we use the common term *plyometrics* to apply to what is actually a system of learning to jump and land. Plyometrics by strict definition is a system of reactive exercises, not just a series of jumps. The program detailed here is really a jump training progression, but for simplicity and familiarity we use the now-generic term *plyometrics* to encompass all phases of the jump training program.

True plyometric drills require the athlete to reduce the time spent on the ground. The athlete learns to minimize the amortization (shock absorption) phase and to respond aggressively to the ground. Although the science behind plyometric training is sound, we have done a poor job of facing the realities and disparities of the human body. We must crawl before we walk and walk before we run.

The same applies to plyometrics. We must learn to jump off the ground and properly land on the ground before we attempt to minimize time spent on the ground. Gravity is the enemy of the large athlete, the young athlete, and the weak athlete, and gravity must be respected when teaching an athlete to jump or when attempting to develop explosive power.

Plyometric training can be controversial. Some experts have cautioned against the initiation of a plyometric program with athletes who do not have a proper leg strength base. In fact, some articles on plyometric training have suggested that an athlete needs to be able to do a back squat with a weight equal to two times body weight before even commencing a plyometric program. In reality, this is a ridiculous recommendation that eliminates nearly 90 percent of athletes. The two-times-body-weight guideline was suggested decades ago as a precursor to beginning high-level plyometrics, but somewhere along the line the concept was incorrectly applied to all plyometric training.

Other authors suggest an 8-week strength phase before commencing a plyometric program. Although this suggestion is slightly more rational, it is still not practical because most athletes train for only 10 to 12 weeks in the off-season. An 8-week strength phase leaves only 4 weeks of plyometric training at most, a period far too short in which to implement a periodized program.

The essential elements of an effective plyometric program are that the exercises are taught in a progressive manner and that progress is based on competence, not on a predetermined timeline. If an athlete cannot move beyond phase 1 jumps, that athlete should stay in phase 1 for an additional two or three weeks before attempting to progress. Don't try to force progress.

Much has been written about plyometric training for athletes. However, very few articles or books have detailed a progressive program that takes into account the need for a system of training that can be applied to a broad range of athletes. Past works on plyometrics by people such as Don Chu, Jim Radcliffe, and Vern Gambetta were outstanding, but not enough has been written that connects our current knowledge of functional training and functional anatomy with the process of how to design and implement a system of plyometric exercises. To begin to understand plyometrics, we must look at the basics of terminology, exercise type, and exercise variables.

Terminology

The language of plyometrics must be universal so that any coach or athlete can view the program of any other coach or athlete and understand the exercises in the absence of photos or video. Discrepancies in terminology were first brought to my attention by Mike Clark of the National Academy of Sports Medicine. Clark pointed out in a 2000 lecture that many coaches currently used names to describe plyometric exercises that were not properly descriptive of the movement. Clark went on to detail the types of exercises and the specific actions:

Jump: double-leg takeoff followed by double-leg landing

Hop: single-leg takeoff, landing on the same foot

Bound: single-leg takeoff, landing on the opposite foot

Skip: single-leg takeoff with two foot contacts

Although these descriptions might be viewed as simple and common sense, I realized I had inadvertently misclassified exercises. We had always referred to double-leg jumps over hurdles as hurdle hops. I believe this confusion in terminology was and still is common among many strength and conditioning and track coaches.

Clark pointed out that "bunnies don't hop, they jump." A matter of semantics or just a minor discrepancy, you say? I thought so too until I received a call from a coach in California who made me realize the potential cost of such "minor discrepancies." The coach in question called me and said, "Boy, are your guys great athletes. I can't get one guy on my team to do those 30-inch hurdle hops your guys do." I quickly realized that my "minor discrepancy" had made this coach try to perform an exercise with one leg that we had been doing with two. He had his athletes hurdle-hopping as the program indicated, while I had mine hurdle-jumping. This is just one example of how lax attention to descriptive terminology or incorrect interpretation of what is described can put athletes at risk of serious injury.

Exercise Categories

After terminology, the next area to examine is the types of jumps, hops, and bounds. I believe this is the major failing of the most popular commercially available anterior cruciate ligament (ACL) injury prevention programs. The two most popular, the Santa Monica PEP program and the Sportsmetrics program, focus almost exclusively on jumps with no emphasis on bounds or hops. The reality is that the mechanism of the ACL tear is most frequently a single-leg hop (actually a redundancy as the term *hop* denotes a single leg) or bound scenario, not a double-leg jump. Doing jumps to prevent injuries that occur in hopping or bounding situations borders on a waste of time.

A sound plyometric program must include a balance of exercises from each terminology category. Much like we balance push and pull in strength training, athletes must perform a balance of jumps, hops, and bounds. In addition, hops must be done both forward and side to side. It should be noted that hopping medially and laterally are entirely different in both the muscles stressed and the injury prevention potential. Medial hops (hops toward the midline) are more difficult and provide much needed stress to the hip stabilizers.

Jump Volume

The number of jumps per session, or jump volume, has most frequently been measured by the number of times the feet contact the ground. A major failing of many plyometric programs is that they require many foot contacts. Our approach is to keep the number of foot contacts deliberately low and gradually increase the intensity of the jumps or hops rather than increasing the volume.

We try to keep the number of foot contacts at roughly 25 per day and 100 per week. Failing to control the number of foot contacts per day and per week is a surefire road to overuse knee injuries.

Intensity

The intensity of plyometric training is difficult to measure and really involves understanding the difference between a program of controlled jump training and a true plyometric program. As previously mentioned, many exercises that we consider to be plyometric in nature are actually simply jumping exercises.

Controlling the intensity of plyometric exercises is based on how gravity is allowed to work on the body. Intensity is increased by either increasing the contribution of gravity or by attempting to change the nature of the amortization phase. This is accomplished either by jumping over an object rather than up onto an object or by introducing an elastic component through a bounce and then a rebound.

Jumps or hops up to a box are the lowest intensity because they involve a strong concentric contraction but minimize eccentric stress by not allowing the body to "in effect" come down. The body is accelerated up to a height but the athlete steps down, effectively negating gravity as an accelerant and a potential stressor.

Chu's early work classified intensity of jumps based on whether they were done in place or covered horizontal distance. Although this early quantification system of in-place, short, and long was state of the art in the 1980s, our increased awareness of the effects of physics on the body led us to a system that I believe better describes the effect and stress of jumps, hops, and bounds. I prefer classifying jumps as gravity reduced (jumps up to a box) or gravity enhanced (jumps over a hurdle) and then moving to semi-elastic jumps and finally true elastic plyometrics.

Early plyometric descriptions did not acknowledge that certain jumps were not actually plyometric in nature. True plyometrics involve an effort to minimize time on the ground and an attempt to enhance reactivity to the ground. In our system these true plyometric exercises are done in the fourth phase. Generally athletes do not exceed 100 foot contacts per week, even in the later phases. What changes is the intensity of the jumps, not the volume.

Frequency

One of the first questions when discussing the frequency of plyometric exercises relates to the National Strength and Conditioning Association's initial position statement on the subject. The NSCA took the stance that plyometrics should be done only twice per week. This has since been amended to read that the same joints should not be worked on consecutive days. (Note: The NSCA takes no position on intensity or volume other than to indicate that depth jumps may be too intense for larger athletes.)

My belief is that plyometrics can be performed up to four times per week but must be divided into linear and multidirectional days. Linear plyometrics involve pure sagittal-plane jumps and hops, while multidirectional plyometrics work in the frontal and transverse planes.

Age and Level of Experience

Another interesting point in the NSCA statement relates to the development of a proper strength base for plyometrics. Unfortunately, no one has defined what that proper strength base is.

In my opinion, strength training and plyometric training can be done concurrently providing common sense is used. The reality is that young athletes begin intense plyometric programs without a strength training base or a required strength level every day. Both gymnastics and figure skating involve intense plyometric activity from very young ages. The key is to manage the effect of gravity on the body.

QUIET, PLEASE!

Good plyometrics are quiet. Failure to land quietly indicates that the athlete lacks eccentric strength and that the exercise is inappropriate. All that may be necessary is to decrease the height of the obstacle involved. Athletes should only jump onto boxes that they can land on quietly and should land in the same position or depth of squat that they took off from. In the same regard, athletes should only jump over objects that allow them to land properly.

PROGRESSION TO PLYOMETRICS

An effective process of readying an athlete's body for plyometric training is to teach jumping and landing skills before introducing what many coaches and athletes would classify as plyometrics. The strength of this type of programming is that it prioritizes injury prevention over power development.

Phases 1 through 3 of this progressive plyometric program are not the true plyometrics that many coaches might recognize. They are actually a series of drills designed to teach jumping skills, to develop the ability to land with great stability, and to introduce the elastic component of jumping. This progression to plyometric training does not introduce true plyometrics until phase 4.

The plyometric drills for each phase are classified as linear drills or lateral drills. One inadvertent failing of many plyometric programs is that the programming is very track and field influenced. Because track and field is purely sagittal, many programs tend to jump or hop only up or forward and neglect the frontal plane that is so important to most team sports.

To be truly functional an athlete must be able to jump, hop, or bound not only forward but to the right and left as well. The influence of track and field and its inherently sagittal nature is felt heavily in the areas of speed and plyometric training.

A quick recommendation for plyometric training equipment: If you are going to buy boxes for your phase 1 plyometrics, spend the extra money and get foam boxes. The new foam boxes not only soften the landing but also prevent injuries caused by missing the box.

Phase 1: Jumps, Hops, and Bounds With a Stable Landing

In a progressive plyometric program, the emphasis of the first phase is on learning to jump and more importantly to land. Athletes should be taught to summate forces using the arms and hips and to land softly. The more softly the athlete lands, the better. Athletes must learn to absorb forces with their muscles, not with their joints.

The purpose of phase 1 is to develop eccentric strength. Think of eccentric strength as the brakes on a moving vehicle. This first phase is the most important and unfortunately the most overlooked and underappreciated phase of plyometric training. Skipping or attempting to abbreviate phase 1 is the main cause of injury. You'll be surprised how poor some elite athletes are at landing.

No matter what performance level an athlete has achieved, she should always begin in phase 1. Whether the athlete is a pro or a middle school student, phase 1 lasts a minimum of three weeks, but coaches and athletes should take as long as they need to in this phase. The goal of phase 1 is to develop stability and the eccentric strength necessary to land. Another way to think of phase 1 is as tendon training.

The following exercises should be done once or twice per week.

▶ BOX JUMP

This linear exercise is the most basic of all the jumping drills. Select a box height that is appropriate for athletic ability. Many athletes want to inflate their egos by using a box that is too high. The coach should not be afraid to choose the box for the athlete if the athlete displays a poor sense of his own jumping ability. For beginners, box height ranges from 4 to 24 inches (10 to 60 cm) depending on the skill level of the athlete. Do three to five sets of 5 jumps, up to 25 jumps total, or in plyometric lingo, 25 foot contacts.

The criteria for evaluating whether the box height is correct are simple.

1. Can the athlete land quietly? If not, then the box is too high.
2. Does the athlete land in the same position that she took off in? If the landing knee bend is significantly deeper than the takeoff knee bend, the box is too high.

The comparison between landing and takeoff is a great suggestion made by Oregon strength coach and plyometrics expert Jim Radcliffe in his lectures and writings. This simple, no-nonsense concept helps coaches determine whether athletes are performing the box jump correctly. The landing position should never be deeper than a half-squat position. See figure 9.2.

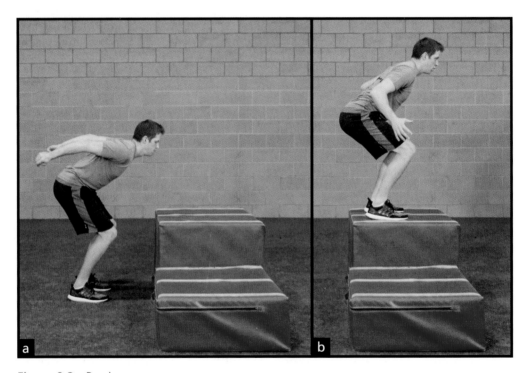

Figure 9.2 Box jump.

THE IDIOT BOX

If you have plyo boxes of either 36- or 42-inch (90 or 105 cm), please put them away. In fact, unless you are training some great athletes, put your 30-inch (75 cm) box away, too.

I have dubbed the big plyo boxes Idiot Boxes because they are used by young men looking to show off. I have begun to refer to such young men as "skin donors." I can tell you something for sure. There was a time when my athletes and I were foolish—just like everyone else—and did these foolish exercises. After coaching a few skin donors, I realized that what mattered was the movement of the center of mass, not the height of the box. I no longer keep a 36-inch box at my facility, but I do have lots of 18-inch (45 cm) and 24-inch (60 cm) boxes and a few 30-inch boxes.

SINGLE-LEG BOX HOP

Even though theory tells us that single-leg box hops are less stressful than single-leg hops over an obstacle, for some athletes we use single-leg hops over a low obstacle (in theory a phase 2 exercise) in place of the single-leg box hop or lateral box hop. Often younger or weaker athletes can be intimidated by the prospect of hopping and landing on a low box, and something like a 6-inch (15 cm) mini-hurdle or even a line on the floor will be less intimidating. With our post-ACL athletes we just use a line on a field to begin our hop progression. Very often a single-leg hop up to even the lowest box can cause some anxiety that results in a missed landing and an injury. We do not worry greatly about gravity here as these become almost "confidence hops."

Use the same technique described for the box jump, but begin with something as low as a 4-inch (10 cm) box. Do three sets of 5 hops per leg, for a total of 15 hops per leg. See figure 9.3.

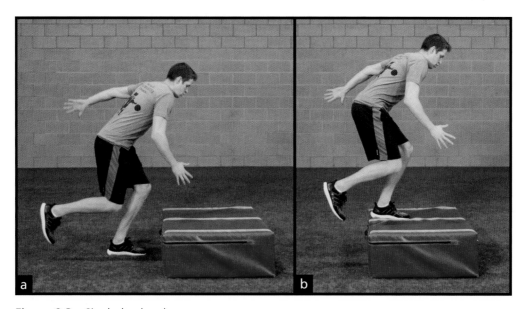

Figure 9.3   Single-leg box hop.

▶ SINGLE-LEG LATERAL BOX HOP

This lateral exercise is also done one day per week. To do the single-leg lateral box hop, hop from the side of a 4-inch (10 cm) box to the top of the box (see figure 9.4). The key is a stable, quiet landing on one leg. Do three medial jumps (toward the midline of the body) and three lateral jumps (away from the midline of the body) per leg. The stabilization forces are markedly different in each case. Do three sets of six jumps (three medial and three lateral) per leg. These can also be done over a very low obstacle, such as a 6-inch (15 cm) mini-hurdle, or even over a line to allow younger or larger athletes to develop more confidence.

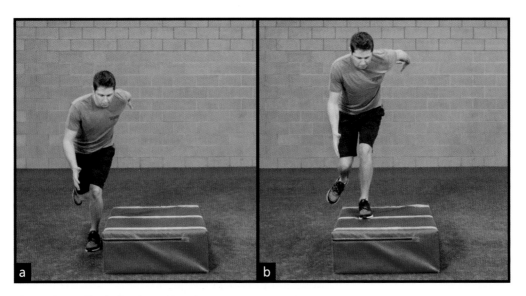

Figure 9.4 Single-leg lateral box hop.

▶ LATERAL BOUND AND STICK

In the original version of *Functional Training for Sports* we used the term *Heiden*, named after legendary speed skater Eric Heiden, to denote a lateral bound. The lateral bound and stick is a basic lateral exercise known by numerous names, including skaters or skate hops. The athlete moves from right to left or left to right and holds the landing for a full second before bounding back to the opposite side. The term *stick* emphasizes that we want the athlete to stick the landing and hold it. Being able to stick a stable landing is critical for all phase 1 exercises. Often athletes ask, "Am I trying to go high or far?" My answer is "both." A good lateral bound is done for a combination of height and distance (see figure 9.5).

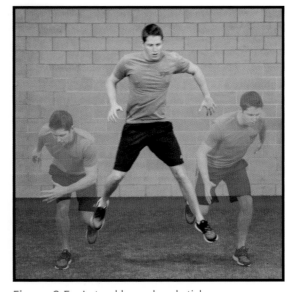

Figure 9.5 Lateral bound and stick.

Do three sets of five bounds on each leg, for 30 total foot contacts.

Phase 2: Jumps, Hops, and Bounds Over an Obstacle

In phase 2 of our plyometric program, gravity becomes a larger component of the drills. Instead of jumping or hopping up on a box or over a very low obstacle as in phase 1, the athlete now jumps over a relatively challenging obstacle, usually a specially designed mini-hurdle. These jumps, hops, and bounds now include both a vertical and a horizontal component. The action of jumping over an obstacle greatly increases the eccentric load on the muscles and tendons.

The goal of a soft landing remains the same, but the addition of the force of gravity greatly increases the eccentric strength demand. Instead of progression coming in the form of more jumps, progression is achieved by increasing the eccentric load of the landings.

The obstacle used is generally a hurdle somewhere between 6 and 30 inches (15 to 75 cm) tall, depending on the type of jump and the athlete's skill level. Al Vermeil, the legendary Chicago Bulls strength and conditioning coach, likes to say, "The bigger the athlete, the smaller the obstacle." This might seem counterintuitive, but Vermeil's statement is brilliant. Six foot 6 inch (198 cm) basketball and football players will struggle mightily with single-leg hops over 6-inch mini-hurdles.

HURDLE JUMP AND STICK

The hurdle jump and stick is a jump over a series of hurdles. The hurdles can range in height from 12 to 30 inches (30 to 75 cm) depending on the skill level of the athlete. Companies such as Perform Better sell molded plastic hurdles in 12-inch, 18-inch (45 cm), and 24-inch (60 cm) sizes. Generally the hurdle height will correspond to the box height used for a properly performed box jump. The key to the hurdle jump is to again finish with a quiet, stable landing (figure 9.6).

Hurdle jumps are a natural, logical progression from the box jump. The big difference is that the body now experiences the acceleration due to gravity on the way down. The concentric action is almost exactly like the box jump, but the eccentric load is drastically increased based on the height of the obstacle and the corresponding movement of the center of mass. Perform three sets of five hurdles, for a total of 15 jumps.

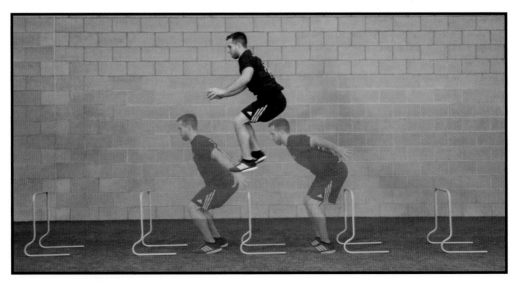

Figure 9.6   Hurdle jump and stick.

▶ SINGLE-LEG HURDLE HOP AND STICK

In the single-leg hurdle hop and stick, the athlete jumps off of and lands on the same leg (see figure 9.7). This drill can be done over lines if landing stability or landing confidence is an issue; however, the goal of advancing from phase 1 to phase 2 is the addition of a hurdle or an increase in hurdle height.

Do three sets of five hops on each leg, for a total of 30 foot contacts.

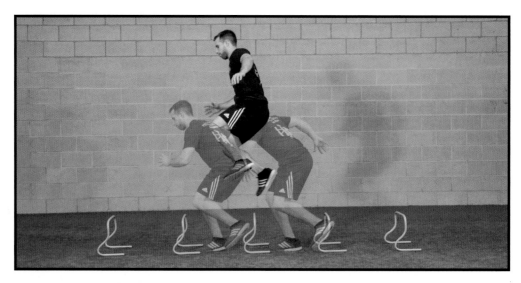

Figure 9.7   Single-leg hurdle hop and stick.

▶ SINGLE-LEG LATERAL HURDLE HOP AND STICK

Use the technique described for the lateral box hop, only over three 6-inch mini-hurdles placed 18 to 24 inches (45 to 60 cm) apart. This is a down and back drill. The athlete hops in a lateral direction over three hurdles placed roughly 18 inches apart, sticking each landing, and then returns by hopping medially over the same three hurdles, sticking the landing for a count of one, one thousand each time (see figure 9.8). The drill can be done over lines if landing stability or landing confidence is an issue. Do three sets of 6 hops on each leg (3 medial and 3 lateral), for 36 hops total.

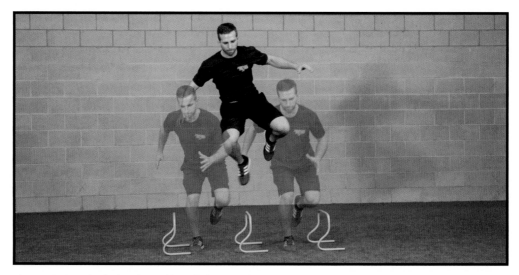

Figure 9.8   Single-leg lateral hurdle hop and stick.

45-DEGREE BOUND AND STICK

The 45-degree bound and stick adds a linear component to the lateral action of the bound as a progression, rather than adding an obstacle. Instead of jumping directly to the side, the push-off is now forward at a 45-degree angle (see figure 9.9). Do three sets of 5 jumps on each leg, for 30 total jumps.

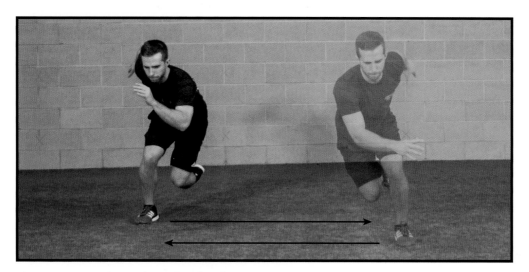

Figure 9.9   45-degree bound and stick.

CAUTION

Another type of plyometric exercise is a decelerative jump in the transverse plan. To visualize this jump, think about taking off in one direction and then turning 90 or 180 degrees before landing. Athletes should take great care when performing transverse-plane jumps and hops. Unfortunately, some authors have recommended transverse-plane exercises that look very much like the injury mechanisms we are trying to avoid.

Phase 3: Phase 2 Exercises With an Additional Bounce

Exercises performed in the third phase begin to resemble what many coaches and athletes consider real plyometrics. The emphasis in phase 3 is on switching from an eccentric contraction to a concentric contraction rather than simply developing eccentric strength by sticking the landings. Although eccentric-to-concentric switching is the essence of plyometric training, most plyometric-related injuries stem from the failure to develop eccentric landing skills.

Phases 1 and 2 laid the essential groundwork for injury prevention and for the later stretch-shortening-cycle work that follows. Phase 3 introduces the stretch-shortening cycle by incorporating a bounce into the drills. The key is to gradually increase the type and amount of stress applied to the muscle and, more importantly, to the connective tissue.

The exercises performed in this phase are identical to those performed in phase 2, but they are now done with a small bounce before the next jump. Stretch shortening is introduced without a drastic change in program. Intensity increases again, but not volume.

HURDLE JUMP WITH BOUNCE

Use the same technique as for the hurdle jump and stick, but instead of sticking the landing add a bounce before the next takeoff.

SINGLE-LEG HURDLE HOP WITH BOUNCE

Use the same technique as for the single-leg hurdle hop and stick, but replace the stable landing with a bounce before the next takeoff. If athletes struggle with this drill, they should resume phase 2 and stick the landing.

SINGLE-LEG HURDLE LATERAL HOP WITH BOUNCE

Use the same technique as for the single-leg lateral hurdle hop and stick, but replace the stable landing with a bounce before the next takeoff. If athletes struggle with this drill, they should resume phase 2 and stick the landing

45-DEGREE BOUND WITH BOUNCE

Use the same technique as for the 45-degree bound in phase 2, but bounce before the next takeoff.

Phase 4: Explosive, Controlled, and Continuous Movements

Phase 4 moves into the realm of what most coaches and athletes consider true plyometrics. In this phase, the emphasis is on reacting to the ground and minimizing ground contact time. If you are wondering, *What took you so long?* the answer is that our approach is to emphasize safety and mastery first. The biggest mistake of an approach that is too conservative is that the early phases are extended longer than necessary.

In phase 4 athletes now strive to minimize time spent on the ground and make an elastic, explosive, but quiet, transition from eccentric to concentric contraction. When great athletes perform plyometrics, one thing is immediately noticeable. You *see* a great deal of explosiveness but *hear* very little. The nervous system and the muscular system do most of the work, with little stress on the joints. This is the goal of the progressive plyometric program.

HURDLE JUMPS (CONTINUOUS)

The athlete performs continuous double-leg jumps over hurdles.

SINGLE-LEG HURDLE HOPS (CONTINUOUS)

As with the linear jumps, the single-leg hops are now continuous, with emphasis on a limited ground contact time.

LATERAL HURDLE HOPS (CONTINUOUS)

Following in the same thought process, the down and back lateral hop action is now also done in continuous fashion.

45-DEGREE LATERAL BOUND (CONTINUOUS)

The 45-degree lateral bound is an aggressive lateral push-off moving from right to left or left to right (see figure 9.10). The athlete performs aggressive abduction to generate lateral power.

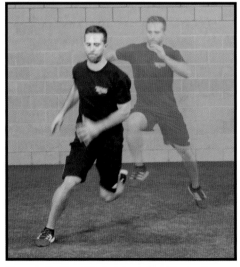

Figure 9.10   45-degree lateral bound.

▶ POWER SKIP

This is a linear drill in which the athlete adds aggressive hip extension to the warm-up skip to gain both height and distance (see figure 9.11).

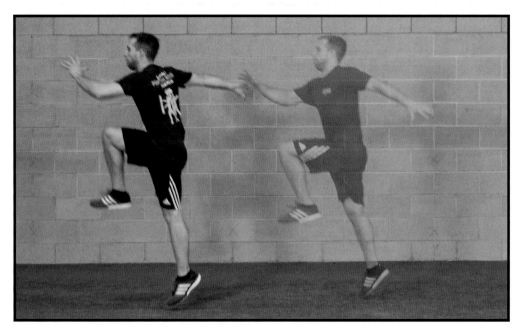

Figure 9.11   Power skip.

PLYOMETRICS AND ACL INJURY PREVENTION

Anterior cruciate ligament tears are approaching near epidemic level in the sports world. Some estimates are as high as 100,000 torn ACLs per year. According to a 2001 lecture by physical therapist Mike Clark, more than 30,000 of these ACL tears are believed to occur in young women who participate in sports such as soccer, basketball, and field hockey. These staggering numbers alone justify addressing ACL injury prevention in any program designed for female athletes.

A number of physical therapy and athletic training groups have begun to sell or promote programs designed for ACL injury prevention. Some are good; some are drastic oversimplifications. A sound ACL injury prevention program needs to focus on two things:

1. Single-leg strength
2. Landing and deceleration skills

Most ACL injuries occur when an athlete who is too weak attempts to land or change direction. Many studies point to predisposing female physiological characteristics such as hip structure, knee structure, and menstrual changes. Coaches, athletes, therapists, and trainers cannot change the bone structure of the athlete or attempt to keep them out of competitive situations at critical points during the menstrual cycle.

We can obsess about why female athletes get ACL injuries more often than male athletes, but our time and energy is better devoted to the things we can change. Coaches and trainers can wring their hands about the physiological predisposition of young women to ACL tears, but this will not change the facts. Girls and young women will continue to play sports in increasing numbers and at higher levels. What can be controlled is the development of single-leg strength, both concentric and eccentric, and the development of landing skills. A combination of strength training and a properly designed and progressed plyometric program is the best ACL injury prevention program in the world.

At MBSC, we tell everyone who will listen that ACL injury prevention is just good training. The idea of an ACL injury prevention program is really just another way to package the idea of good training and sell that idea to a female athlete or her coach. It is amazing how different the response of a female athlete or coach is to an ACL injury prevention program than a strength and power development program.

Regardless of its label, a plyometric program must be properly designed to include hops, jumps, and bounds; be properly planned; and be properly taught. Poorly taught or poorly progressed plyometric exercises can result in patellofemoral joint problems, another area of particular concern for young female athletes.

A plyometric program, and therefore the ACL injury prevention program, should always begin with the phase 1 exercises described earlier. The techniques presented throughout this book are the building blocks of the ACL injury prevention program. Single-leg strength exercises, a proper plyometric program, and a conditioning program that emphasizes changes of direction go a long way toward the prevention of ACL injuries.

The development of strength cannot be overemphasized for young female athletes. They should work through the single-leg strength progression in chapter 6, from split squat to single-leg squat, progressing to the next level when they've mastered the previous one. Most young female athletes need weeks or even months to progress to a true single-leg squat, but the ability to perform the single-leg squat might be the best ACL injury prevention technique available.

While young athletes are developing concentric single-leg strength through strength training, they should simultaneously be developing eccentric strength and landing skills through properly progressed plyometric training. It is critical that plyometric training be properly taught and that all progression be based on competence. The four-phase progressive plyometric program described in this chapter is a fundamental building block of the ACL prevention or rehabilitation program. The initial nine weeks gradually introduces the skills of jumping, hopping, and bounding and more importantly, the stresses of landing.

As mentioned previously, many plyometric experts caution against beginning a plyometric program until the athlete has developed a high level of leg strength, but if their guidelines are followed, young athletes would never gain the benefits of a program of controlled jumping and would miss out on the vital landing skills training that phase 1 plyometrics provide. Not only do you not need a strength base to begin plyometric training, beginning athletes can start with beginning-level plyometrics on day 1. Falling into the trap of "strength base first" only delays the implementation of measures that can prevent ACL tears.

Please remember that to prevent ACL injuries it is important to balance hip-dominant and knee-dominant strength work; to include all the linear and lateral jumping, hopping, and bounding drills; and to follow the progressions. It is critical to work first on landing skills. If only two workout days are available, linear and lateral plyometric work should be done every day.

A progressive plyometric program is one way to improve power output. The sequence in this chapter allows you to safely improve speed, horizontal jumping ability, and vertical jumping ability while decreasing injury potential. The key is to follow the sequence and not skip steps. There is no shortcut to improvement, only shortcuts to injury.

Plyometric training is only one of the three methods proposed for improving power. Plyometrics, medicine ball throws (chapter 7), and Olympic lifting (chapter 10) can be successfully combined to produce great gains in power production.

Remember that more is not better. Do not exceed the recommended number of foot contacts or the recommended number of training days per week. Plyometrics can safely be done up to four days a week if the program is followed as described. Two linear days and two lateral days, each preceded by the corresponding warm-up (chapter 5), will not result in overuse injury if this program is followed. Athletes seeking to safely increase speed, vertical jump, or overall power, or simply to prevent injury, can benefit from the plyometric progressions in this chapter.

Olympic Lifting

Athletes and coaches are always searching for the best and safest methods to develop power. Increased power translates into a faster, more explosive athlete. Evidence continues to mount that explosive lifts, such as the Olympic lifts and their variations, may be the best methods to rapidly improve power output.

The downside is that Olympic lifting requires a great deal of teaching and constant supervision. Many coaches have added Olympic lifting to their programs because of the significant evidence for the benefits; unfortunately, some of these same coaches are not able or willing to teach their athletes proper technique. More recently coaches have begun to use Olympic lifts as high-repetition challenges instead of for power development. We are in a period of hugely increased popularity and exposure for Olympic lifting, but often what we see is akin to watching someone attempt to pound nails with a screwdriver.

The end result of poorly taught, poorly implemented, or unsupervised Olympic weightlifting is often injury. When injuries occur, the blame is often placed on the exercises when the blame should be laid squarely on the shoulders of the coach or the trainer. The key is to think of Olympic lifting as a tool—a powerful tool that can both help and hurt. I like to use the analogy of a chainsaw. A chainsaw can help you cut down a tree, but it shouldn't be used by those with no experience.

Let's begin with a basic premise. Anyone who is uncomfortable with performing or teaching the Olympic lifts should not use them. Get your high-velocity power development work from medicine balls, kettlebell swings, and plyometric exercises.

The key to developing a safe and effective training program is learning to balance what is great in theory with what becomes great in practice. Before adding any explosive movements to a program, coaches must know how to teach the movements, and athletes must learn how to perform them with great technique. Don't be concerned about weight; worry about technique. Remember that you have your hands on a powerful tool.

With that said, Olympic lifting is great functional training. It is done standing and uses almost every muscle in the body in an explosive, coordinated fashion. Large amounts of work can be done in a short period of time after the techniques are mastered. The disadvantages are the needs to teach and coach constantly and the need to be concerned with technique over weight.

Almost all the young athletes at our facility are taught to Olympic lift regardless of sport, unless they have a history of back injury. Adults generally are not Olympic lifters in our system. Adult posture and limitations don't tend to mix well with the Olympic lifts. Baseball players, tennis players, and swimmers also refrain from explosive overhead movements such as the snatch so as to avoid excessive stress on the rotator cuff. Our athletes have an injury rate near zero for supervised Olympic lifts done from a position with the bar above the knees and for the appropriate number of reps. Never use Olympic lifting as a high-repetition endurance activity, but always as a low- to medium-repetition power development activity.

WHY WE OLYMPIC LIFT

Olympic lifting enhances athleticism, develops eccentric strength, and most importantly is fun.

Athleticism

Although Olympic lifting has been shown to have excellent effects on total-body power, increasing power outputs might be the fourth most important reason we Olympic lift. The number one reason we do Olympic lifts is for the effect on coordination and athleticism. I don't know if there is anything more beautiful to watch in the weight room than a well-performed Olympic lift.

Thirty years of experience tells me that the best athletes are also the best Olympic lifters. Coaches might ask themselves if this is a chicken and egg scenario. Are better athletes better Olympic lifters, or do Olympic lifts make you a better athlete? I am not completely sure, but based on what I have observed, heard, and read, I believe Olympic lifting enhances athleticism. I have compared Olympic lifting to tumbling in relation to Olympic lifting's ability to develop athletic ability. I love that an athlete has to perform a jump (the concentric part of the lift) and then navigate a moving object to create the receiving position (the eccentric portion, or the catch).

Eccentric Strength

The number two reason to Olympic lift is to develop eccentric strength. Pulling a weight is one thing. Actually catching and decelerating that same weight is another. Teaching an athlete to produce a powerful concentric contraction and to then catch and decelerate a moving object *might* be the most difficult and beneficial skill that one can do in the weight room. It also might be the best injury prevention work you can do. Learning to not only produce force but to also absorb force and decelerate load is a critical skill in contact sports.

I happen to think there is tremendous injury prevention value in the eccentric strength developed in the catch portion of the Olympic lifts. In sport, injuries often come while absorbing contact, not while delivering a blow. This rapid eccentric component is not present in any exercise besides the Olympic lifts, which makes them of particular benefit to the muscles around the shoulder girdle. In my years in hockey and football, shoulder separations and concussions were rare. I think Olympic lifting played no small part in that.

Fun

Fun? Yes, fun. Olympic lifting is fun. Some athletes learn to enjoy the grind of attempting to lift a heavy load. However, I don't think many people would describe a heavy set of squats or deadlifts as fun. Athletes seem to enjoy Olympic lifts much more. In fact, I always believed Olympic lifts were the great equalizer in the weight room. In sports such as football, the smaller, more explosive athlete rarely competed with his larger teammates in the bench press and the squatting movements, but in the Olympic lifts, the skilled athlete could often outlift a heavier, larger teammate. This was both rewarding and fun.

LEARNING TO OLYMPIC LIFT

The easiest way to learn the Olympic lifts is from the hang position. In this position, the bar is not lifted from the floor and in fact is always kept above the knees (see figure 10.1). The hang position eliminates a great deal of the lower back stress often associated with the Olympic lifts and allows athletes of any size to start learning in very similar, joint-friendly positions. Any athlete can become a great technician from the hang position. Conversely, many athletes will have difficulty learning the Olympic lifts from the floor.

Not all athletes possess the physiological characteristics that make great competitive Olympic weightlifters (good biomechanical lever system, mesomorphic body type, great hip flexibility). In fact, the very qualities that make a good basketball player or rower make a poor competitive weightlifter.

I have never been a fan of cleaning from the floor. In fact, I don't think in 30 years I have ever had an athlete do it. In my mind, Olympic lifts are for power. To improve starting strength, load the bar in the deadlift. If the goal is to improve power, then my choice would be Olympic lifts done from a hang above the knees.

The key in any programming decision is to choose the right tool for the right job. The initial pull from the floor is simply a deadlift that gets the bar into the proper position to perform the hang clean. An athlete who begins an Olympic lift from the floor is, in effect, choosing the wrong tool for the job.

The objective of any training program is to become a better athlete in a specific sport, not to become a competitive Olympic weightlifter (unless that is your sport). Olympic weightlifting should always be the means to an end, not an end itself. EXOS coach Denis Logan said it best when he said we want to make "great athletes that are good weightlifters." What does that mean? It means we see Olympic lifting for what it is—a tool to make great athletes.

Olympic lifts and their variations primarily develop power and athleticism. Although the Olympic lifts develop impressive musculature, this should not be the primary objective. The objective is not to just move a weight but to move a weight in a fast, powerful, and athletic manner. The Olympic lifts are intended primarily to train the nervous system and secondarily to develop the muscular system.

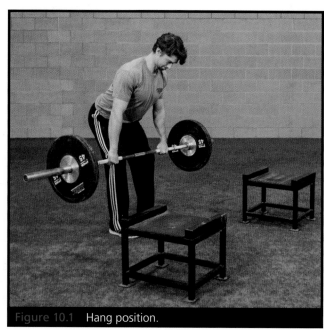

Figure 10.1   Hang position.

GUIDELINES FOR PERFORMING THE OLYMPIC LIFTS

Following are a few guidelines for learning the Olympic lifts.

- Think safety first. Be conscious of the surroundings. Use a lifting platform if one is available. The platform says "keep back," much like caution tape.
- Practice proper technique. This is simple. If it doesn't look right, it probably isn't. The objective of Olympic lifting is not just to move the bar from point *A* to point *B*. The objective is to move the bar quickly and in a technically correct manner from point *A* to point *B*. Once you compromise on this point, you have failed as an Olympic lifter or as a teacher of Olympic lifts.
- Emphasize speed of movement over weight on the bar. Most of the technical mistakes made in learning the Olympic lifts are the result of one thing: *too much weight*. The battle is between ego and common sense. Your best correction is often the simplest and most obvious one: reduce the weight.

Anyone with common sense and the ability to recognize some fundamental positions can learn to clean and snatch.

There may be no single correct way to teach the Olympic lifts. Experts will disagree about many points. There is, however, a simple method we have used with great success to teach athletes in sports from football to field hockey. Remember that your goal is not to produce Olympic weightlifters. The goal is to use Olympic lifting as a tool to make better athletes. Don't get caught up in designing or duplicating a program created for Olympic weightlifters; design a program for athletes to develop power using Olympic lifts and their variations as a portion of their training.

MASTERING THE KEY OLYMPIC LIFTING POSITIONS

Learning the main Olympic lifting positions is a four-step process.

Step 1: Hands-Free Front Squat

It is important to be proficient in the front squat before learning the clean. At MBSC this is the only time we teach front squats with the Olympic bar. The ability to front-squat affects the understanding of the catch portion of the hang clean because the bar is "caught" in a quarter front squat.

Start with the bar resting on the deltoids (muscles that cover the shoulders), with the arms extended out in front (see figure 10.2). The hands are deliberately not on the bar. This step begins to teach the athlete to rack the bar properly and

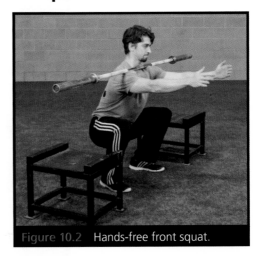
Figure 10.2   Hands-free front squat.

to carry the bar on the shoulders, not on the wrists or in the hands. Most complaints associated with the hang clean result from not catching the bar properly. Don't skip this step; it is critical.

Step 2: Clean-Grip Front Squat

Do not use a cross-over grip in the front squat (see figure 10.3). Athletes must be able to execute a proper front squat to be able to properly catch a clean. This is not a strength lift for us but rather a teaching tool designed to teach an athlete how to properly catch a hang clean.

An athlete having trouble with proper squat technique may have inadequate mobility in the hips and ankles. The optimal way to stretch for the squat is to sit in the full-squat position, place the elbows on the inner sides of the knees, and push the knees out over the toes while arching the back (see figure 10.4).

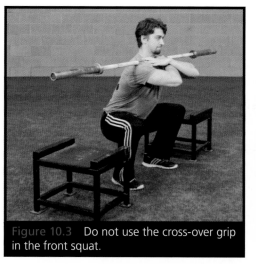

Figure 10.3   Do not use the cross-over grip in the front squat.

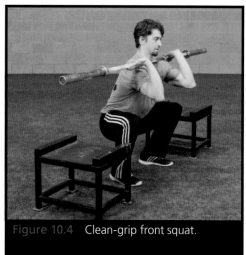

Figure 10.4   Clean-grip front squat.

Step 3: Start Position for the Clean and Snatch

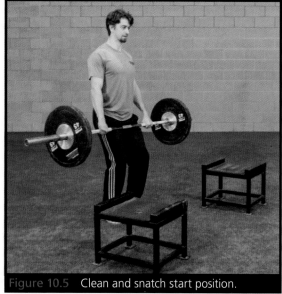

Figure 10.5   Clean and snatch start position.

This is the basic pulling position. Stand with the feet shoulder-width apart, knees slightly bent, chest slightly behind the bar, wrists curled under, arms straight, and elbows turned out (see figure 10.5). This is a change from how the initial position was taught in the original version of *Functional Training for Sports*. Credit here goes to Olympic lifting coach Glenn Pendlay. Rather than teaching an athlete to get the chest over the bar by sliding the bar down the thighs, Pendlay recommends simply bending the knees and keeping the chest slightly behind the bar. This change makes it easier for athletes to execute the simple beginner's jump and catch that comes later. Instead of hinging forward and trying to get the chest over the bar, the athletes simply bend the knees. In this position the chest will be just over the bar or slightly behind the bar. Bending the knees also causes a slight hip flexion. From here the athlete has a better chance of immediate success. The Pendlay technique, as I like to call it, was the first change we had made in our teaching progression in more than 20 years. One thing I am proud of is that we are not so married to our own methods that we miss opportunities to improve.

Step 4: Overhead Support Position

This position is used for the snatch finish, push jerk or push press finish, and overhead squat. Practice supporting the bar overhead with the arms extended. The wrists should be locked, the head slightly forward, the bar over the back of the head, and the legs bent slightly (see figure 10.6).

Remember to perform all Olympic lifts from the hang position (bar above the knees). This is a simple and safe position that can be used easily by athletes of all body dimensions. Larger, taller, or inflexible (i.e., most) athletes have difficulty learning to clean from the floor. Don't listen to so-called experts who insist you must clean from the floor. Remember in athletics Olympic lifting is a tool for power development, not a sport.

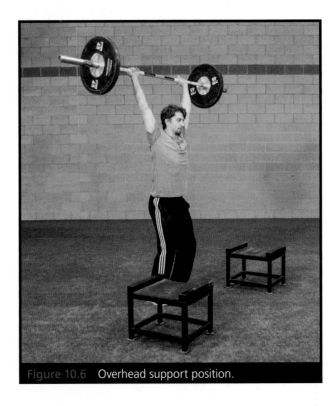

Figure 10.6   Overhead support position.

MASTERING THE HANG CLEAN AND CLOSE-GRIP SNATCH

Step 1: Review how to properly pick up and put down the bar.

Whenever the bar is picked up or put down the back should be arched and tight. This may seem simple, but many injuries are caused by improperly picking up and putting down the bar.

Step 2: Review the hands-free front squat. Learn to control the bar on the deltoids.

This position *must* be learned first. Progress to a clean-grip front squat to establish flexibility in the wrists, shoulders, and elbows.

Step 3: Review the start position.

- Wrists curled under
- Arms straight
- Back arched
- Shoulders slightly behind the bar

Step 4: Bend the knees.

As mentioned, this is a major change.

Step 5a: Perform the hang clean.

With a slightly wider than shoulder-width grip, jump, shrug, and catch in the front squat position (see figure 10.7). Grip is relaxed, with the elbows up and pointed either straight ahead or 45 degrees to the side.

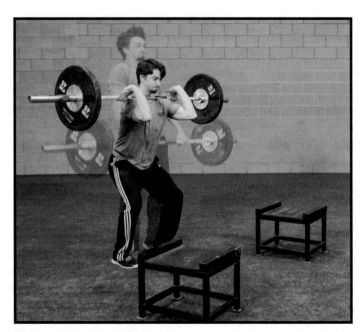

Figure 10.7 Hang clean.

Step 5b: Perform the close-grip snatch.

The close-grip snatch uses a grip identical to that of the clean. The wide grip generally taught for the snatch is discouraged, as its only true purpose is to allow the athlete to lift more weight. Review the overhead support position with a shoulder-width grip. Keep the bar over the back of the head, knees bent, and back arched (see figure 10.8). While executing the snatch, visualize trying to throw the bar up to hit the ceiling. I often tell athletes just that. My best teaching cue is "Try to throw the bar up and hit the ceiling, but don't let go." You'll be amazed how quickly that one cue teaches the snatch.

Note: Snatches are easier to teach and to learn than cleans. Coaches and athletes may initially be intimidated but will grasp the lift quickly. The ability to learn the hang clean can often be limited by upper body flexibility, but there will be no such problem with the hang snatch.

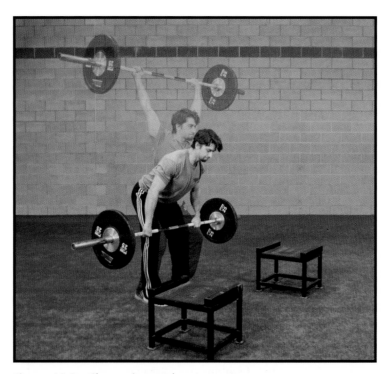

Figure 10.8   Close-grip snatch.

Step 6: Return the bar properly to the blocks.

Keep the back flat and tight.

TEACHING CUE REVIEW

Cues for the start position:

Eyes are straight ahead.

Chest is up.

Back is arched.

Arms are long and loose at the elbows.

Wrists are curled under. (This is key to keeping the bar close to the body.)

Knees are bent. (Remember that the shoulders should be just over the bar or slightly behind the bar in the start position.)

Cues for the pull:

Jump and shrug.

Jump and sit.

Jump and get the elbows up (for the pull).

Cues for the catch (clean only):

Sit under the bar.

Keep the elbows up. Note: One out of 30 athletes is actually not flexible enough to get the elbows up; 29 out of 30 say they can't.

Keep the hips back.

USING LIFTING STRAPS

When advanced lifters begin to struggle to hold the bar and seem to be concentrating as much on grip as on the lift, we introduce lifting straps. The bottom line is we never want to limit lower body power because of a lack of grip strength. That makes no sense. We do not teach a hook grip. We do not tell them they need to concentrate. We do not tell them they need additional carries to work on grip. We teach them to use straps.

Our primary goal is power development. Straps undoubtedly help that. Learn how to properly use straps and how to teach an athlete to use them. They may regress initially, but they will thank you later.

ALTERNATIVES TO OLYMPIC LIFTING

What if you don't want to or can't Olympic lift but still want to make gains in lower body power in the weight room? Jump squats, kettlebell swings, and even single-leg or single-arm versions of the hang clean and hang snatch may be the answer.

Note: Very few of our adult clients Olympic lift. The popularity of CrossFit has led many adults to attempt to learn them, but I believe most adults have undergone too much postural change to become efficient Olympic lifters. Adults are much better off with jumps, swings, and throws for power. From an injury prevention standpoint, it is a mistake to try to teach Olympic lifting to the average adult.

▶ SINGLE-ARM DUMBBELL SNATCH

The single-arm dumbbell snatch is a great alternative for athletes looking to get the value of the Olympic lifts with lower loads on the low back. This exercise is best geared to athletes because the shoulder loads will be substantial. Most athletes will dumbbell snatch more than 50 percent of what they are capable of snatching. The hips and legs are still producing force but are transferring that force into one dumbbell, through one arm.

Step 1: Learn the start position for the dumbbell snatch.

This is still the basic pulling position. Stand with the feet slightly wider than shoulder-width apart, knees slightly bent, dumbbell between the knees, chest over the dumbbell, wrist curled under, arm straight, and elbow turned out.

Step 2: Perform the single-arm dumbbell snatch.

From the start position with the dumbbell between the knees, jump, shrug, and catch the dumbbell in the overhead support position (see figure 10.9). I have found it helpful to cue the athlete with "You should try to hit the ceiling with the dumbbell" and "Pull it as if you were going to let go."

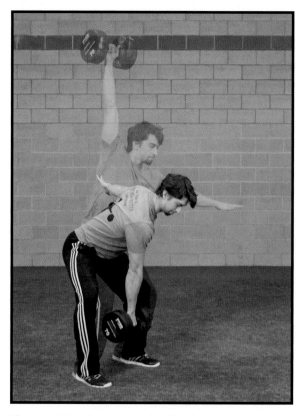

Figure 10.9   Single-arm dumbbell snatch

SINGLE-LEG CLEANS AND SNATCHES

Many coaches believe this is a crazy idea and some consider it outright blasphemy. However, for athletes with back issues or other injury problems, the single-leg versions of the clean and snatch may be just what the doctor ordered.

Start with a load that is 50 percent of what you would normally use in the hang clean or hang snatch. Single-leg Olympic lifting can be a great way to take advantage of cross transfer (using the opposite limb to produce a strength effect in the injured limb) as athletes return from lower body injury and also a great way to keep an athlete returning from a back injury engaged and involved in the program. As crazy as this sounds, give them a try.

Step 1: Learn the start position for the single-leg clean or single-leg snatch.

Everything about the upper body stays exactly the same. The major change is that the athlete is now standing on one leg.

Step 2: Perform the single-leg clean or single-leg snatch.

From the start position, jump, shrug, and catch exactly as you would in the bilateral version (see figure 10.10). These are quite fun for athletes and can really reengage an athlete coming back from injury.

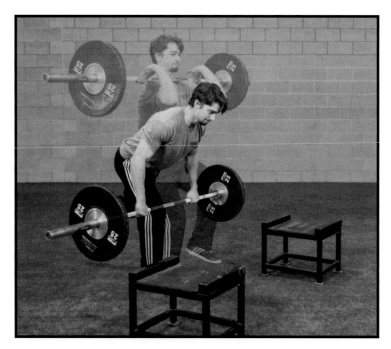

Figure 10.10   Single-leg clean or single-leg snatch.

JUMP SQUATS

Jump squats have been popular for years with European track-and-field athletes and can be a great alternative to Olympic lifts. Jump squats provide a great deal of the hip power that many athletes seek from Olympic lifting and are perfect for athletes who have reservations about technique or athletes with shoulder or back problems that prevent them from Olympic lifting.

To perform the jump squat, simply jump from a position slightly above full-squat depth. Beginners can land and stabilize between jumps, and more advanced athletes can eventually utilize a plyometric response off the floor.

An important issue for jump squats is load selection. Older guidelines recommend using a percentage (most often 25 percent) of the athlete's back squat 1RM as a load. This method of loading is extremely flawed, as it does not take into account the athlete's body weight. The following example illustrates this point.

If athlete A has a 1RM in the back squat of 500 pounds (227 kg) and athlete B also has a 1RM of 500 pounds, then both athletes would use 125 pounds (57 kg) for jump squats using the guideline of 25 percent of back squat 1RM. Now assume that athlete A weighs 200 pounds (90 kg) and athlete B weighs 350 pounds (160 kg). Obviously, athlete A has a strength-to-body-weight ratio far superior to that of athlete B. Loading athlete A with 125 pounds may be reasonable, but athlete B, who weighs 350 pounds, would probably have difficulty executing a technically sound jump squat with an additional external load of 125 pounds. In fact athlete B may have difficulty performing jump squats with just body weight because of his relatively poor strength-to-body-weight ratio. Instead of a 1RM percentage, the following formula is suggested.

[(Squat + body weight) $\times$ .4] – body weight = jump squat weight

Athlete A: [(500 + 200) $\times$ .4] – 200 = 80

Athlete B: [(500 + 350) $\times$ .4] – 350 = –10

The example actually produces a negative number for athlete B. This shows that the 350-pound athlete gets sufficient loading from performing jump squats with body weight but would be overloaded by at least 125 pounds if he followed the simplistic percentage of 1RM guideline. For athlete A, a load of 80 pounds (36 kg) is sufficient.

Consider the total weight an athlete can squat as a combination of body weight and the weight on the bar, and use this number to calculate the load for jump squats. This guideline can be used by both weaker athletes looking to develop power or by larger athletes.

KETTLEBELL SWINGS

Kettlebells have exploded in popularity over the last decade. When our first edition was published in 2004 there was no mention of kettlebells. Now the kettlebell swing has become a mainstream exercise and one of our go-to exercises for power development in those that either do not want to Olympic lift or should not Olympic lift. Although volumes have been written about how to do a proper swing, it is a relatively easy exercise to teach and to program.

But a couple of cautionary notes are worth making. All athletes should be able to touch their toes before deadlifting or swinging. And athletes should master the kettlebell deadlift before starting to perform swings.

MASTERING THE KETTLEBELL SWING

Step 1: Learn the start position for the swing.

This is still the basic pulling position. Stand with the feet slightly wider than shoulder-width apart, hips flexed, back arched, knees slightly bent, kettlebell between the feet but about a foot (30 cm) in front, chest over the kettlebell, wrists curled under, arms straight, and elbows turned out.

Step 2: Perform the kettlebell swing.

From the start position with the kettlebell out in front, think about hiking a football. A good swing starts with that hiking action and the kettlebell staying high. Dan John likes to say, "Attack the zipper." The outside of the forearms should make contact with the inside of the thighs, and the kettlebell should almost smack you in the butt. From here think hip extension.

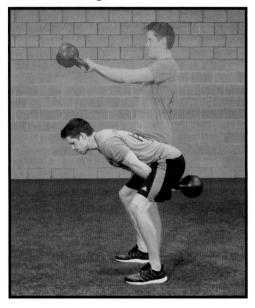

Figure 10.11   Kettlebell swing.

With long arms and a tight low back, snap the hips forward. Think of the arms as just connectors to the kettlebell. The kettlebell should rise no higher than shoulder level and should get to that level from the aggressive hip action, not from any upper body contribution.

Common Mistakes

- *Squatting the swing.* The swing is a hip-dominant movement with lots of hip flexion and very little knee bend. Bad swingers squat their swings.
- *Using the arms.* The swing is not an upper body exercise. Move the kettlebell with a snap of the hips.
- *Rounding the back.* This is a huge mistake and probably the most potentially dangerous.

Explosive lifting can be fun, safe, and challenging when done correctly and supervised aggressively. Work on developing great technique, and put less emphasis on the amount of weight lifted. Choose your candidates carefully, and avoid Olympic lifts with adults. This process will lead to improvements in power and athleticism that you might not have thought possible.

Whether you choose to develop hip and leg power through Olympic lifting, by performing jump squats, or through kettlebell swings, using external loads to train for leg and hip power can be the fastest way to achieve gains in speed or jumping ability. The beauty of Olympic lifts, jump squats, and swings is that the athlete can develop power without necessarily developing muscle bulk. The emphasis is on the nervous system, not the muscular system, making this an excellent training method for athletes such as figure skaters, wrestlers, and gymnasts. Many athletes and coaches have the mistaken impression that explosive lifting is for football players only. This could not be further from the truth. Olympic lifting and its variations are suitable for athletes in all sports and of all sizes and should be of particular interest to athletes looking for total-body strength without increases in size.

ROLE OF THE ROCK

First, let me explain the evolution of the rock, the shift, or the scoop depending on your choice of name. What is clearly evident in both the hang snatch and hang clean is that something happens as a good athlete initiates the explosive phase of the lift, and it happens naturally.

Our athletes have been taking advantage of rotary hip action for more than 20 years. We didn't initially teach this weight shift. In fact, it just happened as the loads got heavier. Better lifters soon realized that trying to hang clean a heavy weight from a dead stop is a difficult task. The better athletes naturally began to rock or weight shift. They also began to hang clean a lot of weight. For a few years I simply let the lift evolve and at numerous points in the '80s and '90s had more than 30 football players hang cleaning more than 300 pounds (136 kg). Not bad for a I-AA football team.

A few years later I made the foolish mistake of listening to my critics, who said that rocking or weight shifting was wrong and that we needed to stop. I started vigorously coaching my athletes to be perfectly still before the explosive part of the lift. I essentially forbade them from rocking or weight shifting. The results were simple and obvious. Our numbers dropped and dropped a lot. One of my athletes actually came up to me and said, "Nice job, you've managed to make us all weaker." His hang clean max had dropped from 370 to 340. (Please note: This player's vertical jump increased 12 inches in four years from 20 to 32 inches.) I was conflicted. I just wanted to do what was best for my athletes. No one was injured rocking, and everyone could lift more weight. I began to do some analysis of the situation and came to the conclusion that rocking was a normal part of both athletics and of Olympic weightlifting.

I can remember reading Carl Miller's *Olympic Lifting* training manual in the late 1970s and reading about what he referred to as "double knee bend." My first reaction was to think it was impossible. However, after watching good Olympic weightlifters on video, it became obvious that it was not only possible but that every great lifter did it. Watch some video in slow motion and you'll see. In order for the bar to clear the knees, the hips and knees extend. After the bar clears the knees, the knees flex or rebend to move the hips into position. In the jump portion of the lift the knees extend again. The cycle is extend–flex–extend. This has been referred to as rocking, scooping, or double knee bend. In any case, it is real and it happens.

The rock you see in Olympic lifts is this same action. Weight shifts back to the heels, knees extend. Weight shifts forward, knees flex. Hips explode, and hips and knees extend. What we are doing is what every athlete does to create maximal explosive power. Watch the vertical jumps at the NFL Combine. What do you see? Rocking, prestretch, weight shift. Call it what you want, but it is the best way to produce a powerful maximal effort.

We routinely have female athletes cleaning 135 pounds (61 kg) for reps, and the majority of my hockey players hang clean between 250 (113 kg) and 320 (145 kg). Healthy athletes, great clean numbers, great speed improvement, great vertical jump. So, am I wrong? I don't think so. As Lee Cockrell says in *Creating Magic*, what if the way we always did it was wrong?

Performance Enhancement Programs

Sport-specific programming is one of the greatest misconceptions in athletics today. The notion that each sport needs its own individual program is fundamentally flawed. The majority of team sports and even many individual sports have similar general needs. All rely on speed and power, with strength as the underlying base. The development of speed, strength, and power does not and should not vary greatly from sport to sport.

Most of the best strength and conditioning coaches in the country use very similar programs to train athletes across a wide range of sports. Very rarely do coaches encounter athletes who are too strong, too fast, or too efficient in lateral movement. Think about it this way: Is a fast baseball player in any way different from a fast football or soccer player? As a coach, would you develop speed for baseball differently from speed for football or soccer?

Coaches may argue that the testing is different, but that is not the question. The *training* would probably not differ. What probably matters most is the athlete's ability to accelerate in a 10-yard area and to decelerate rapidly, not her ability to perform the favored test for the particular sport. The same idea applies to strength. If a baseball player wanted to get stronger, would the process be any different from that for making a football player stronger? I do not believe so. For sports such as baseball, tennis, and swimming, the program might take into account the high stresses on the shoulder and thus reduce the amount of overhead lifting, but most other elements would remain the same. Strength is strength.

There is not one way to get stronger that makes more sense for one sport than another, and there is not any one speed development program that makes more sense for one sport than another. What is important are the similarities, not the differences. This is the beauty of functional training. Usable strength and usable speed are developed in a sensible fashion.

What may be more sport specific is the amount of time dedicated to the development of strength, not the methods used. Programs can range from a two-day in-season program, to a three-day program for a high school athlete during the school year, to the four-day programs we follow in the summer or with our professionals in the off-season. Tell me how much time you have and I'll tell you which program to use. The ideal is a four-day program, but schedules and logistics often don't allow for using the four-day programs.

All programs begin with a preparation period and follow a set recipe. Extending the analogy between a cook and a chef at the beginning of chapter 4, I consider a training plan to be a recipe, not a menu. You can't add or subtract items without affecting the final outcome. So, not coincidentally, the recipe that follows is very similar to the chapter sequence of this book.

Step 1: Foam rolling

Step 2: Static stretching

Step 3: Mobility, activation, and dynamic warm-up

Step 4: Power work, medicine ball throws, plyometrics, and speed work

Step 5: Power and strength work in the weight room

Step 6: Conditioning

The sample programs in this chapter take a phase-by-phase approach to preparation and warm-up skills and a phase-by-phase approach to strength and power in the weight room. This is consistent with all the material leading up to this point, and with the underlying philosophy of training with a purpose and using programs that will achieve that aim.

DESIGNING THE POWER AND STRENGTH PROGRAM

Ideally all strength training programs begin with power development via explosive exercises or Olympic lifts. In other words, the fast stuff gets done first. The interval between sets is allocated to core training, mobility exercises, or both to make the best possible use of time.

After the explosive lifts are completed, athletes typically perform a pair of strength exercises, usually the major lifts for that specific day. Again, this pair of strength exercises may have a core exercise or a mobility exercise added between them to make good use of rest time. We call a pair of strength exercises with mobility or core in between a tri-set.

For us, programming is all about density, and density is basically how much work we can do per hour. In our programs what others view as rest time is instead used for active stretching, mobility work, or core work.

The remaining exercises are done in another tri-set or in mini-circuit style. This means they are either done as already described or done one after another, from exercise one down to exercise four. This tri-set or mini-circuit contains what we view as auxiliary lifts or accessory movements. They are generally done for two or three sets or circuits, with one minute or less of rest between sets. The exception to the rule is the two-day programs. Both tri-sets contain major exercises for that day.

As mentioned already, the major sport-specific differences are not primarily in the strength training programs but instead are in the development of the energy systems for particular sports. The exception is overhead athletes and overhead sports. Baseball, swimming, tennis, and volleyball are examples of overhead sports that might have slightly altered strength programs.

Conditioning programs need to be much more sport specific than strength programs. The strength programs presented are applicable to a broad range of sports, but the conditioning programs may be more specific to a single sport or group of sports.

Program Components

There are the 9 essential components of a well-designed functional strength program. All of these are covered in detail in the preceding chapters. The components are utilized and combined based on the number of training days available. As the number of training days decreases from four to three to two, the decisions about priority become increasingly difficult. In two-day programs things become very simple: an explosive exercise, a push, a knee-dominant exercise, a pull, and a hip-dominant exercise. In a four-day program certain components may be done twice per week. In a two-day program each component is addressed only once.

1. Explosive power development—most often Olympic lifts, but plyometric work, swings, or jump squats can be substituted (see chapters 9 and 10)
2. Bilateral hip-dominant exercises—generally trap-bar deadlifts (see chapter 6), but kettlebell sumo deadlifts and goblet squats may also be used
3. Single-leg knee-dominant exercises—single-leg squats, split squats, and variations (see chapter 6)
4. Unilateral hip-dominant exercises—straight-leg deadlifts and variations (see chapter 6)
5. Core work—antiextension, antirotation, antilateral flexion (see chapter 7)
6. Horizontal presses—bench presses, incline presses (see chapter 8)
7. Vertical presses—dumbbell or kettlebell overhead presses (see chapter 8)
8. Horizontal pulls—rows and variations (see chapter 8)
9. Vertical pulls—chin-ups and variations (see chapter 8)

The key to a properly designed functional training program is combining these categories without overemphasizing or underemphasizing any particular component.

Two-day workouts follow the same thought process as three- and four-day workouts and generally begin with an Olympic movement such as a hang clean, hang snatch, or dumbbell snatch. Incline presses can be used as a compromise between supine pressing and overhead pressing.

Strength Program Phases

We have used the Poliquin undulating model of three-week phases, which alternate between higher volume (accumulation phases) and lower volume with heavier loads (intensification phases), with great success. Three weeks tends to work well with most off-season programs because you can use four phases that are 3 weeks long during a 12-week off season.

Phase 1 is the base phase. Poliquin refers to this as an accumulation phase, meaning the athlete accumulates more volume during this period. This may also be referred to as an anatomical adaptation phase or as a hypertrophy phase. We start with two sets of 8 to 10 reps in week 1 to acclimate our athletes with relatively lower volumes, progressing to three sets in weeks 2 and 3. Olympic lifting is performed for five reps.

Phase 2 makes strength development the focus and is referred to as an intensification phase. In other words, intensity increases while volume decreases (the weight goes up and the reps go down). We may use sets of three for bench presses, chin-ups, and Olympic lifts, with sets of five for our lower body strength exercises, such as rear-foot-elevated split squats and single-leg straight-leg deadlifts. In this phase the volume for exercises decreases from 24 reps (three sets of 8) to between 9 (three sets of 3) and 15 (three sets of 5). Intensities move from the 70 percent range into the low 80 percent range.

Phase 3 is a second accumulation phase, but methods can vary. We may use complex training (pairing a strength exercise with a power exercise), eccentric emphasis (accumulating time and volume with lower reps), or a modified program of three sets (10-5-20) to work across a range of spectrums. In any case, during phase 3 the total volume of work again increases, moving back toward 24 reps total volume.

Phase 4, for most sports, is a strength–endurance phase focusing on slightly higher reps that begins to prepare the athlete for the preseason practices to come. But it can be another lower-rep strength phase for some athletes involved in high-absolute-strength sports such as football. Complex training may be used in this phase if it has not been used in the previous phase.

We have used this model very successfully for a long time and continue to fine-tune it.

Sample Strength Programs

Please note that all programs should be preceded by a thorough dynamic warm-up session. Allot 60 to 90 minutes for each training session to cover preworkout soft tissue work, stretching, warm-up, and strength work.

All the workouts shown are copies of spreadsheets used. In Excel, if the athletes' max lifts are known, they can be used to calculate loads. Max weights are the key data that allow the sheet to calculate bench loads, split-squat loads, and clean loads. These max weights are only relevant in that they produce the actual spreadsheet numbers.

To use the chart, simply read across from left to right. Perform the lift listed, with the given weight and number of reps.

Four-Day Programs

Four-day programs (see tables 11.1-11.5) are preferred for off-season training for most sports because coaches can easily combine all the elements needed for strength development, speed development, and conditioning. Few compromises are necessary to address all the critical variables. The four-day workout allows inclusion of additional core work or prehabilitation exercises that might not fit into a two- or three-day workout.

Table 11.1 Sample Four-Day Workouts

Day 1	Day 2	Day 3	Day 4
Explosive/Olympic Antiextension core	Pair Horizontal Push Upper Mobility	Explosive/Olympic Antiextension Core	Pair Incline Push Upper Mobility
Pair Hip dominant Vertical pull	Pair Vertical Push Upper Mobility/ Stability	Pair Knee dominant Vertical pull	Pair Horizontal Push Hip Mobility
Tri set Knee dominant Horizontal Pull Antirotation Core	Tri set Core-Misc Antirotation Core Loaded Carry	Tri set Hip dominant Horizontal Pull Antirotation Core	Tri set Core-Misc Antirotation Core Loaded Carry

Table 11.2 Summer Lift Phase 1

Day 1	Week 1 reps	Week 2 reps	Week 3 reps	Day 2	Week 1 reps	Week 2 reps	Week 3 reps
Hang clean progression	5	5	5	Bench press	8	8	8
Wk1 hang clean from pos. 1	5	5	5		8	8	8
Wk2 hang clean from pos. 1	5	5	5		—	8	8
Front plank progression	2×20 sec	2×25 sec	2×30 sec	Spiderman pos. lat stretch	2×5 breaths	2×5 breaths	2×5 breaths
Trap bar deadlift	8	8	8	Half-kneeling alt overhead press	8	8	8
	8	8	8		8	8	8
	—	8	8		—	8	8
Chin-up	8	8	8	Supine floor slide	8	8	8
	8	8	8		8	8	8
	—	8	8		—	—	—
Bottoms-up split squat or one-leg squat	8 each side	8 each side	8 each side	Push-up progression	8	8	8
	8 each side	8 each side	8 each side		8	8	8
	—	8 each side	8 each side		8	8	8
Dumbbell row	8	8	8	TK push-pull	8	8	8
	8	8	8		8	8	8
	—	8	8		—	8	8
In-line chop	2x8	2x8	2x8	Suitcase carry	25 yards each side 2×	25 yards each side 3×	25 yards each side 3×

(continued)

Table 11.2 Summer Lift Phase 1 *(continued)*

Day 3	Week 1 reps	Week 2 reps	Week 3 reps	Day 4	Week 1 reps	Week 2 reps	Week 3 reps
Hang clean progression	5	5	5	Dumbbell incline bench	8	8	8
Wk1 hang clean from pos. 1	5	5	5		8	8	8
Wk2 hang clean from pos. 1	5	5	5		—	8	8
Front plank progression	2×20 sec	2×25 sec	2×30 sec	*Spiderman pos. lat stretch*	2×5 breaths	2×5 breaths	2×5 breaths
Rear-foot-elevated split squat	8 each side	8 each side	8 each side	Push-up progression	8	8	8
	8 each side	8 each side	8 each side		8	8	8
	—	8 each side	8 each side		8	8	8
Ring row	8	8	8	*Squat holds*	6	6	6
	8	8	8		6	6	6
	—	8	8		—	—	—
Dumbbell single-leg deadlift	8 each side	8 each side	8 each side	Quarter get-up	3 each side	4 each side	4 each side
	8 each side	8 each side	8 each side		3 each side	4 each side	4 each side
	—	8 each side	8 each side		—	4 each side	4 each side
X-pull-down	8	8	8	TK antirotation press out	8	8	8
	8	8	8		8	8	8
	—	8	8		—	8	8
In-line lift	2×8	2×8	2×8	Farmer carry	25 yards each way 2×	25 yards each way 2×	25 yards each way 2×
Conditioning	**Week 1**	**Week 2**	**Week 3**	**Conditioning**	**Week 1**	**Week 2**	**Week 3**
Sled march weights:				Sled crossover weights:			
				1 mile time:			

Table 11.3 Summer Lift Phase 2

Day 1	Week 1 reps	Week 2 reps	Week 3 reps	Day 2	Week 1 reps	Week 2 reps	Week 3 reps
Hang clean *Progress to pos. 2 if ready*	3	3	3	Bench press	5	5	5
	3	3	3		5	5	5
	3	3	3		5+	5	5
	—	—	—		—	5+	5+
Hard-style front plank	2×20 sec	2×25 sec	2×25 sec	*Spiderman pos. lat stretch*	2×5 breaths	2×5 breaths	2×5 breaths
Trap bar deadlift	5	5	5	Standing overhead press	5	5	5
	5	5	5		5	5	5
	5+	5	5		5	5	5
	—	5+	5+		—	—	—

Day 1	Week 1 reps	Week 2 reps	Week 3 reps	Day 2	Week 1 reps	Week 2 reps	Week 3 reps
Chin-up	5	5	5	*Supine floor slides*	10	10	10
	5	5	5		10	10	10
	5	5	5		—	—	—
One-leg squat	6	6	6	Push-up progression	10	10	10
	6	6	6		10	10	10
	6	6	6		10+	10+	10+
Dumbbell row	10	10	10	Half-kneeling push-pull	8	8	8
	10	10	10		8	8	8
	10	10	10		8	8	8
In-line iso hold chop	2×8	2×8	2×8	Suitcase carry	25 yards each way 3×	25 yards each way 3×	25 yards each way 3×

Day 3	Week 1 reps	Week 2 reps	Week 3 reps	Day 4	Week 1 reps	Week 2 reps	Week 3 reps
Hang clean (65-75%) *progress to pos. 2 if ready*	5	5	5	Dumbbell incline bench	5	5	5
	5	5	5		5	5	5
	5	5	5		5	5	5
	—	—	—		—	5+	5+
Hard-style front plank	2×20 sec	2×25 sec	2×25 sec	*Spiderman pos. lat stretch*	2×5 breaths	2×5 breaths	2×5 breaths
Rear-foot-elevated split squat	5	5	5	Push-up progression	10	10	10
	5	5	5		10	10	10
	5+	5	5		10+	10+	10+
	—	5+	5+		—	—	—
Ring row	10	10	10	*Toe touch squat with medicine ball*	6	6	6
	10	10	10		6	6	6
	10	10	10		—	—	—
Dumbbell single-leg deadlift	5	5	5	Get-up	3 each side	4 each side	4 each side
	5	5	5	*1st roll to elbow*	3 each side	4 each side	4 each side
	5	5	5	*To high bridge*	3 each side	4 each side	4 each side
X-pull-down	10	10	10	Half-kneeling antirotation hold	3×20 sec	3×25 sec	3×25 sec
	10	10	10				
	10	10	10				
In-line isometric hold lift	2×8	2×8	2×8	Farmer carry	25 yards each side 2×	25 yards each side 2×	25 yards each side 2×

Conditioning	Week 1	Week 2	Week 3	Conditioning	Week 1	Week 2	Week 3
Sled march weights:				Sled crossover weights:			
150 times:				1-mile time:			

Table 11.4 Summer Lift Phase 3

Day 1	Week 1 reps	Week 2 reps	Week 3 reps	Day 2	Week 1 reps	Week 2 reps	Week 3 reps
Hang clean	3	3	3	Bench press *complex with medicine ball bench*	5	5	5
	3	3	3		3	3	3
	3	3	3		3+	3+	1+
	3	3	3		—	—	—
Stability ball roll-out	3×6	3×8	3×8	*Spiderman pos. lat stretch*	2×5 breaths	2×5 breaths	2×5 breaths
Trap bar deadlift *complex with continuous hurdle jump*	5	5	5	Standing overhead press	5	5	5
	5	5	5		5	5	5
	5	5	5+		5	5	5
Chin-up *complex with medicine ball slam 3×10*	3	3	3	*Supine floor slide*	10	10	10
	3	3	3		10	10	10
	3+	3+	3+		—	—	—
One-leg squat	5	5	5	Push-up progression	10	10	10
	5	5	5		10	10	10
	5	5	5		10+	10+	10+
Dumbbell row	5	5	5	Dynamic push-pull	8	8	8
	5	5	5		8	8	8
	5	5	5		8	8	8
Dynamic chop	3×10	3×10	3×10	Suitcase carry	25 yards each way 3×	25 yards each way 3×	25 yards each way 3×

Day 3	Week 1 reps	Week 2 reps	Week 3 reps	Day 4	Week 1 reps	Week 2 reps	Week 3 reps
Hang clean (65-75%)	5	5	5	Dumbbell incline bench *complex with medicine ball bench*	5	5	5
	5	5	5		3	3	3
	5	5	5		3+	3+	3+
Stability ball roll-out	3×20 sec	3×25 sec	3×25 sec	*Spiderman pos. lat stretch*	2×5 breaths	2×5 breaths	2×5 breaths
Rear-foot-elevated split squat *complex with continuous hurdle hops*	5	5	5	Push-up progression	10	10	10
	3	3	3		10	10	10
	3+	3+	3+		10+	10+	10+
Ring row *complex with medicine ball slam 3×10*	10	10	10	*Toe touch squat with medicine ball*	8	8	8
	10	10	10		8	8	8
	10	10	10		—	—	—

Day 3	Week 1 reps	Week 2 reps	Week 3 reps	Day 4	Week 1 reps	Week 2 reps	Week 3 reps
Dumbbell single-leg deadlift	6	6	6	Get-up	2+2	2+2	2+2
	6	6	6	*1st roll to elbow*	2+2	2+2	2+2
	6	6	6	*To high bridge full get-up*	2+2	2+2	2+2
Dumbbell row	5	5	5	Standing antiro-tation hold	3×25 sec	3×25 sec	3×25 sec
	5	5	5				
	5	5	5				
Dynamic lift	3×10	3×10	3×10	Farmer carry	25 yards each way 3×	25 yards each way 3×	25 yards each way 3×
Conditioning	**Week 1**	**Week 2**	**Week 3**	**Conditioning**	**Week 1**	**Week 2**	**Week 3**
Sled march weights:				Sled crossover weights:			
300 times:				1-mile time:			
150 times:							

Table 11.5 Summer Lift Phase 4

Day 1	Week 1 reps	Week 2 reps	Week 3 reps	Day 2	Week 1 reps	Week 2 reps	Week 3 reps
Hang clean	3	3	3	Bench press *complex with medicine ball bench*	5	5	5
	3	3	3		3	3	3
	3	3	3		3+	3+	1+
	3	3	3		—	—	—
Stability ball roll-out	3×6	3×8	3×8	*Spiderman pos. lat stretch*	2×5 breaths	2×5 breaths	2×5 breaths
Trap bar deadlift *complex with continuous hurdle jumps*	5	5	5	Standing over-head press	5	5	5
	5	5	5		5	5	5
	5	5	5+		5	5	5
Chin-up *complex with medicine ball slam 3×10*	3	3	3	*Supine floor slide*	10	10	10
	3	3	3		10	10	10
	3+	3+	3+		—	—	—
One-leg squat	5	5	5	Push-up progression	10	10	10
	5	5	5		10	10	10
	5	5	5		10+	10+	10+
Dumbbell row	5	5	5	Dynamic push-pull	8	8	8
	5	5	5		8	8	8
	5	5	5		8	8	8
Dynamic chop	3×10	3×10	3×10	Suitcase carry	25 yards each way 3×	25 yards each way 3×	25 yards each way 3×

(continued)

Table 11.5 Summer Lift Phase 4 *(continued)*

Day 3	Week 1 reps	Week 2 reps	Week 3 reps	Day 4	Week 1 reps	Week 2 reps	Week 3 reps
Hang clean (65-75%)	5	5	5	Dumbbell incline bench *complex with medicine ball bench*	5	5	5
	5	5	5		3	3	3
	5	5	5		3+	3+	3+
Stability ball roll-out	3×20 sec	3×25 sec	3×25 sec	*Spiderman pos. lat stretch*	2×5 breaths	2×5 breaths	2×5 breaths
Rear-foot-elevated split squat *complex with continuous hurdle hops*	5	5	5	Push-up progression	10	10	10
	3	3	3		10	10	10
	3+	3+	3+		10+	10+	10+
Ring row *complex with medicine ball slam 3×10*	10	10	10	*Toe touch squat with medicine ball*	8	8	8
	10	10	10		8	8	8
	10	10	10		—	—	—
Dumbbell single-leg deadlift	6	6	6	Get-up	2+2	2+2	2+2
	6	6	6	*1st roll to elbow*	2+2	2+2	2+2
	6	6	6	*To high bridge full get-up*	2+2	2+2	2+2
Dumbbell row	5	5	5	Standing antirotation hold	3×25 sec	3×25 sec	3×25 sec
	5	5	5				
	5	5	5				
Dynamic lift	3×10	3×10	3×10	Farmer carry	25 yards each way 3×	25 yards each way 3×	25 yards each way 3×
Conditioning	**Week 1**	**Week 2**	**Week 3**	**Conditioning**	**Week 1**	**Week 2**	**Week 3**
Sled march weights:				Sled crossover weights:			
300 times				1-mile time:			
150 times							

Three-Day Programs

Three-day programs (see tables 11.6-11.8) are slightly more difficult to design than four-day programs because they provide 25 percent less training time. Three days is the minimum time recommended for off-season training. The exceptions are programs for athletes who have less need for absolute strength or athletes such as figure skaters, gymnasts, and swimmers who already devote a large part of their time to training and would have difficulty complying with a three-day program. In most team sports, three days should be considered the minimum amount of off-season training.

In a three-day program you can still balance the key components. Fewer compromises are needed than for a two-day program, although some are still necessary. In three-day programs, athletes still begin with an explosive exercise every day and perform a primary pair followed by a tri-set.

Table 11.6 Sample Three-Day Workouts

Day 1	Day 2	Day 3
Explosive/Olympic Antirotation core Antiextension core	Explosive/Olympic Antirotation core Antiextension core	Explosive/Olympic Antirotation core Hip mobility
Pair Hip dominant Vertical pull	Pair Horizontal press Knee dominant, single	Pair Horizontal press Knee dominant
Tri-set Knee dominant Overhead press Loaded carry	Tri-set Hip dominant, single Horizontal pull (row) Loaded carry	Tri-set Hip dominant Horizontal pull Antirotation core

Table 11.7 Fall Lift Phase 1: New Player

Day 1	Week 1 reps	Week 2 reps	Week 3 reps	Day 2	Week 1 reps	Week 2 reps	Week 3 reps
Clean *(Focus on speed and follow teaching progression)*	5 5 5	5 5 5	5 5 5	Kettlebell swing *(Teach Kettlebell deadlift first)*	10 10 10	10 10 10	10 10 10
Incline chop	2×8 each side	2×10 each side	2×12 each side	*Incline lift*	2×8 each side	2×10 each side	2×12 each side
Front plank	2×25 sec	2×30 sec	2×35 sec	*Front plank*	2×25 sec	2×30 sec	2×35 sec
Trap bar deadlift or kettlebell deadlift	8 8 8	8 8 8	8 8 8	Eccentric bench press 3 sec eccentric/1 sec pause *Baseball: dumbbell bench 3×8*	8 8 8	8 8 8	8 8 8
Chin-up (slow eccentric) *Regression: TRX row*	Max Max − 1 Max − 1	Max Max Max − 1	Max Max Max − 1	Eccentric rear-foot-elevated split squat	8 each side 8 each side 8 each side	8 each side 8 each side 8 each side	8 each side 8 each side 8 each side
Push-up progression *Regression: standing cable press*	8 8 8	8 8 8	10 10 10	Suspension row	8 8 8	8 8 8	8 8 8
Goblet squat	5 5 5	5 5 5	5 5 5	Goblet squat	8 8 8	8 8 8	8 8 8
TK antirotation press	3×8 each side	3×10 each side	3×12 each side	Seated external and internal rotation *(ball or light dumbbell)*	2×8	2×10	2×12
Supine band pull-apart: 2×8, 10, 12							

(continued)

Table 11.7 Fall Lift Phase 1: New Player *(continued)*

Day 3	Week 1 reps	Week 2 reps	Week 3 reps	GOALS
Clean	5	5	5	1:
	5	5	5	
	5	5	5	
Farmer carry	2×turf	3×turf	3×turf	
Front plank	2×25 sec	2×30 sec	2×35 sec	
Half-kneeling alternating dumbbell press	8 each side	8 each side	8 each side	2:
	8 each side	8 each side	8 each side	
	—	8 each side	8 each side	
Dumbbell single-leg deadlift or reaching	8 each side	8 each side	8 each side	INJURIES TO NOTE:
	8 each side	8 each side	8 each side	
	—	8 each side	8 each side	
Dead stop dumbbell row *Regression: cat–cow*	8 each side	8 each side	8 each side	
	8 each side	8 each side	8 each side	
	—	8 each side	8 each side	COMMENTS:
Half get-up	3 each side	4 each side	5 each side	
	3 each side	4 each side	5 each side	
	—	4 each side	5 each side	
Eccentric slide-board leg curl with half roller *Regression: hip lift*	8	8	8	
	8	8	8	

Table 11.8 Fall Lift Phase 1: Returning Player

Day 1	Week 1 reps	Week 2 reps	Week 3 reps	Day 2	Week 1 reps	Week 2 reps	Week 3 reps
Clean (*Focus on speed; follow teaching progression*)	5	5	5	Kettlebell swing (*Teach kettlebell deadlift first*)	10	10	10
	5	5	5		10	10	10
	5	5	5		10	10	10
Incline chop	2×8 each side	2×10 each side	2×12 each side	*Incline lift*	2×8 each side	2×10 each side	2×12 each side
Front Plank	2×25 sec	2×30 sec	2×35 sec	*Front plank*	2×25 sec	2×30 sec	2×35 sec
Trap bar or kettlebell deadlift	8	8	8	Eccentric bench press 3 sec eccentric/1 sec pause; *baseball: dumbbell bench 3×8*	8	8	8
	8	8	8		8	8	8
	8	8	8		8	8	8
Chin-up (Slow eccentric) *Regression: TRX row*	Max	Max	Max	Eccentric rear-foot-elevated split squat	8 each side	8 each side	8 each side
	Max − 1	Max	Max		8 each side	8 each side	8 each side
	Max − 1	Max − 1	Max − 1		8 each side	8 each side	8 each side
Push-up progression *Regression: standing cable press*	8	8	10	TRX Row	8	8	8
	8	8	10		8	8	8
	8	8	10		8	8	8
Single-leg squat	8	8	8	Goblet squat	8	8	8
	8	8	8		8	8	8
	8	8	8		8	8	8
TK antirotation press	3×8 each side	3×10 each side	3×12 each side	Seated external and internal rotation (*ball or light dumbbell*)	2×8	2×10	2×12

Supine band pull apart: 2×8, 10, 12

Day 3	Week 1 reps	Week 2 reps	Week 3 reps	GOALS
Clean	5	5	5	**1:**
	5	5	5	
	5	5	5	
Farmer carry	2×turf	3×turf	3×turf	
Front plank	2×25 sec	2×30 sec	2×35 sec	**2:**
Half-kneeing alternating dumbbell press	8 each side	8 each side	8 each side	
	8 each side	8 each side	8 each side	
	—	8 each side	8 each side	

(continued)

Table 11.8 Fall Lift Phase 1: Returning Player *(continued)*

Day 3	Week 1 reps	Week 2 reps	Week 3 reps	INJURIES TO NOTE:
Dumbbell single-leg deadlift or reaching	8 each side	8 each side	8 each side	
	8 each side	8 each side	8 each side	
	—	8 each side	8 each side	
Dead stop dumbbell row *Regression: cat–cow*	8 each side	8 each side	8 each side	
	8 each side	8 each side	8 each side	
	—	8 each side	8 each side	COMMENTS:
Half get-up	3 each side	4 each side	5 each side	
	3 each side	4 each side	5 each side	
	—	4 each side	5 each side	
	—	8 each side	8 each side	
Eccentric slide-board leg curl with half roller *Regression: Hip lift*	×8	×8	×8	
	×8	×8	×8	

Two-Day Programs

Two-day programs (see table 11.9) are the most difficult to design. They are generally used during the season or in sports that do not require a lot of absolute strength. I recommend two-day programs only for in-season workouts. Please note that all programs should be preceded by a thorough dynamic warm-up session. Allot 60 to 90 minutes for each training session to cover preworkout soft tissue work, stretching, warm-up, and strength work.

The difficulty with two-day programs is attempting to train all the essential areas in only two sessions. Compromises must be made.

Table 11.9 Sample Two-Day Workouts

Day 1	Day 2
Explosive/Olympic Core	Explosive/Olympic Core
Pair 1 Bilateral hip dominant Horizontal press (supine)	Pair 1 Unilateral knee dominant Horizontal press (incline)
Pair 2 Vertical pull Unilateral knee dominant	Pair 2 Horizontal pull (row) Unilateral hip dominant

DEVELOPING CONDITIONING PROGRAMS

Conditioning for sport is constantly developing and changing. Coaches and trainers have made huge advances in their understanding of the physiology of sports and in designing programs that stress the appropriate energy systems. Although many programs now use work-to-rest ratios that are more appropriate for team sports, not enough programs address change of direction as a vital component of sport conditioning.

A comprehensive performance enhancement conditioning program must factor in all you have learned throughout this book about functional training. Programs should be designed with some simple concepts in mind:

- Utilize the minimal effective dose concept, beginning with body weight when practical.
- Design a program that can be completed in the allotted time. Think about how long each set will take and how much rest to allow between sets. A good guideline is about 16 to 20 sets in a one-hour workout.
- Design a workout that addresses all the key components, or as many as practical in the time available.
- Design a workout that prepares an athlete to play a sport, not a workout that mimics one of the strength sports (bodybuilding, powerlifting, Olympic lifting). Simulating a strength sport may be the largest mistake in program design.

Good conditioning program design takes time and thought. Don't waste valuable training time with worthless exercises. Always go for the most bang for the buck. Most single-joint exercises do not work a movement pattern but instead work one joint action in one plane. Exercises such as lunges and split squats can be used to develop single-leg strength, balance, and flexibility. This three-pronged benefit is the key to good exercise selection.

The areas of conditioning that now need to be developed are muscular specificity and movement specificity. All the programs illustrated in this chapter address change of direction as a key component of the conditioning process. The ability to tolerate the muscular forces generated by accelerating and decelerating and the ability to adapt to the additional metabolic stress caused by acceleration and deceleration are the real keys to off-season conditioning. Deficiencies in these components are often why athletes describe themselves as not being in "game shape."

Most athletes have trained by running, or worse, riding a set distance in a set amount of time with no thought to the additional stresses provided by having to speed up and slow down. Athletes frequently are injured in training camp settings in spite of following a prescribed conditioning program to the letter. This is usually due to following a conditioning program that ignores the vital components of the conditioning process:

1. Acceleration
2. Deceleration
3. Change of direction

Developing the Conditioning Base

Our philosophy toward developing a conditioning base intentionally leaves out the term *aerobic*. As stated in chapter 2, the concept of aerobic base may be fine in the simplistic sense, but the pursuit of an aerobic base through steady-state exercise can be counterproductive. The key to any conditioning program should be to *prepare the athlete to play the sport*.

Asking athletes in sprint-dominant sports (most team sports) to develop a base conditioning level through long, steady-state activity can lead to negative physiological changes at the cellular level and to negative muscular changes in tissue quality, tissue length, and joint range of motion. In addition, steady-state conditioning exposes the muscles and joints to potential overuse injury. To prepare properly, athletes need to accelerate and decelerate, and the muscles and joints need to move in a motor pattern that is similar to the pattern used at top speed.

With this said, the obvious question is, How do you develop a conditioning base without jogging? The answer in my mind is that you work backward. Instead of beginning a conditioning program with multiple bouts of 30 to 40 minutes of jogging or cycling, begin with small amounts of extensive tempo running, gradually increasing the amount and correspondingly the time. Our conditioning workouts initially may take only 10 minutes, but they are preceded by up to 20 minutes of dynamic warm-up. The end result is 30 minutes of elevated heart rate with an emphasis on dynamic flexibility and proper motor patterns. Contrast this with 30 minutes of range-limited jogging to develop the aerobic base.

It is important to mention that extensive tempo running is neither sprinting nor jogging; rather, it is periods of striding interspersed with periods of walking. Athletes stride 30 to 100 yards or meters, depending on the facility size, and walk 30 to 40 yards or meters after each stride. Athletes should begin with approximately 6 to 8 minutes of tempo runs and elevate the heart rate through a combination of striding and walking. In general, athletes should never jog or revert to the short-stride motor pattern that is often implicated in loss of flexibility.

The tempo runs are done once per week. From tempo runs athletes progress to shuttle runs that emphasize acceleration, deceleration, and change of direction. The shuttle runs are also done once per week. Initially, 150-yard (150 m) shuttle runs are done on a 25- or 50-yard course. This allows the athletes to change direction while accelerating and decelerating.

In the first week of shuttle runs the total distance covered is decreased (from approximately 1,000 yards of tempo running to 750 yards of shuttle running) to compensate for the increased muscular stress of the shuttle runs. Shuttle-run distances are then increased by either 10 to 20 percent per week (about 150 yards).

It's important to note that the use of a 25-yard course results in increased muscular stress by doubling the number of changes of direction and changes in speed. However, many facilities do not have access to the 60 yards of straightaway space needed to run at 50-yard intervals.

Using a progression of tempo runs to shuttle runs allows the athlete to

1. develop a base while maintaining the appropriate muscle lengths and

2. achieve a level of conditioning to safely and effectively perform stops and starts, which are part of so many sports.

Customizing Conditioning for a Sport

In general, conditioning programs must be sport specific in terms of these characteristics:

- *Time.* In chapter 2 we discussed analyzing the needs of a sport. Conditioning programs should not be designed to allow the athlete to pass an arbitrary conditioning test but to prepare the athlete to participate in the sport itself.

- *Movement.* Conditioning programs should incorporate changes of direction. Injuries most often occur in acceleration and deceleration. Often athletes are injured not because they are out of shape but because they are poorly prepared. One minute of straight-ahead running on a track and one minute of stop-and-start shuttle running are drastically different, both muscularly and metabolically.

- *Motor pattern.* Conditioning must incorporate the pattern of a sprint (i.e., the stride pattern must be similar to sprinting). To properly condition the hip flexors and hamstrings (the muscles most often injured in the preseason), the athlete must aggressively extend and recover the hip. Consider that a six-minute mile is run at the speed of an eight-second 40-yard dash. No wonder many athletes who think they are prepared often injure themselves.

- *Movement emphasis.* The workouts are arranged so that on lateral movement days, conditioning has a lateral movement emphasis. This means that two days per week, conditioning is done on the slide board, regardless of the sport. The slide board provides repeated frontal-plane acceleration and deceleration. There is no better complement to running than the slide board.

Linear and Lateral Training

Tempo running and shuttle running are used on linear days, whereas slide-board work is done on lateral days. The slide board is an excellent method of conditioning that meets a number of needs in all sports.

The slide board was made popular by Olympic speedskater Eric Heiden in the 1980s. Speedskaters have been using the slide board for decades to develop

FRANCIS'S HIGH–LOW CONCEPT

Another key component to conditioning programs involves how hard to work. There has been backlash in recent years about coaches working athletes too hard, with too much change-of-direction running. An example is running timed shuttle runs on every conditioning day. Legendary sprint coach Charlie Francis espoused a simple high–low approach years ago that has been adopted by thousands of coaches. What Francis effectively said was to make your conditioning workouts either above 90 percent effort or under 80 percent effort. Too much hard work from a conditioning standpoint can be detrimental. As a result we tend to have one hard conditioning workout a week and two or three days in the 70 percent effort range. Those "low" days can be tempo runs, slide-board workouts, or bike workouts.

skating-specific conditioning and mechanics when ice surfaces are unavailable. However, other athletes and coaches have been slow to recognize the value of the slide board as part of their off-season and preseason training. Continued improvement in slide-board design has resulted in some durable boards that can be used by athletes at all levels. Boards that are adjustable from 7 feet to 10 feet (2 to 3 m) are now available.

The slide board may offer the most bang for the buck of any functional conditioning tool. No other piece of equipment can do all of the following:

- Place the athlete in a sport-specific position (for almost all sports)
- Positively stress the abductor and adductor muscles for injury prevention
- Allow athletes to work in groups of three or four on one piece of equipment
- Provide functional conditioning in an interval format for three or four athletes with no adjustments (e.g., seat height) for under $,1000

All athletes regardless of sport (unless they are rowers) should perform lateral movement conditioning two out of four days per week. The slide board may be the best, most cost effective conditioning mode available except for actual running.

The slide board may also be the most important training device available for hockey. Until the advent of the slide board, hockey players were relegated to off-season training on an exercise bike or on the track. Although both running and biking can increase aerobic capacity and anaerobic endurance, there is little similarity to the motion of skating. The slide board provides a highly hockey-specific method for doing work-capacity workouts. In addition, it allows athletes to improve skating technique. Athletes can easily self-correct by placing the board in front of a large mirror and viewing their knee flexion, knee extension, and ankle extension while training. Training with a slide board during the off-season can help hockey players improve work capacity and skating technique for in-season competition.

The slide board also drastically reduces all athletes' chances of incurring preseason groin injuries. The motion of the slide board works the abductor, adductor, and hip flexor muscles, which does not occur on a bike or on any commercially available climber. In addition, the slide board works on the direct lateral pattern that is used in any change of direction and in top-speed skating. When combined with a program of plyometrics and sprints, the slide board is a major tool for improving speed.

Combining the slide board with a weight vest offers another sport-specific mode of hockey and football training. Only football and ice hockey involve the additional weight of equipment as a variable in the conditioning process. For the last half of the summer conditioning program, football and hockey players at our training facility train with 10-pound (5 kg) weight belts on the slide board to begin acclimating them to the weight of their sport's equipment. Some coaches minimize the impact of the equipment, but consider how different the results would be if athletes were tested in a mile run and then retested three or four days later while wearing a 10-pound weight vest or belt. Equipment weight is an important factor in some sports and should be considered in conditioning programs designed for those sports. Not adding weight to the body when conditioning for sports such as hockey and football is foolish.

Seasonal Conditioning Considerations

Many athletes now participate in sport year round, and this must be factored into the off-season conditioning programs. Basketball players, soccer players, and hockey players tend to be on the court, field, or ice year round, as are many others. This means these athletes might do non-weight-bearing conditioning such as an elliptical machine or a stationary bike for additional conditioning. In designing the conditioning program, think about whether you are adding stress to an already stressed system.

Programs that force athletes to increase speed, decrease speed, and change direction drastically reduce the incidence of early-season groin and hamstring injuries and better prepare the athletes for the demands of an actual game or event. However, if the athletes are engaging in these activities daily as a sport-specific workout, alternative activities that complement rather than repeat the movements and stressors of playing the sport should be considered.

Sport-Specific Conditioning Considerations

Strength and conditioning coaches and sports coaches always need to keep in mind what physical capabilities make athletes outstanding in their sport. With that in mind, these are my recommendations.

Football

Football is one of the few sports that is not year round and requires a good off-season interval running program. Football players should run, not bike or do circuits. Football practice is demanding, and running before the start of preseason practices better prepares the athletes to meet that challenge. I believe the big increase in NFL injuries correlates directly to fewer organized team activities and thus a reduction in off-season conditioning days and running.

Baseball

Baseball is unique because it requires on-demand speed but not a large fitness requirement. For this reason, athletes must perform both short sprints for speed and sprint intervals for conditioning. Baseball players will ramp up rapidly in spring training because games come quickly, so adhering to a sprint-interval conditioning program in the off-season is essential.

Baseball at the professional level may be the most unique sport in that you have three very distinct groups of players: position players who play every day, starting pitchers who pitch every fifth day, and relief pitchers who pitch more frequently but with significantly less volume. All have different conditioning requirements. Position players further break down into infielders and outfielders, and both groups have different speed and conditioning requirements. This bears no resemblance to baseball at the lower levels, high school and below, where players play multiple positions. In either case, baseball players must work on speed development to prepare for the demands of the game and on conditioning development to ensure health throughout the season

Pitchers have often done distance running with the mistaken impression that it will develop the endurance necessary to throw 100-plus pitches. Game observation shows a pattern of 10 to 12 pitches per inning followed by about 15 minutes' rest. So since those 100 pitches are often thrown over the course of three to four hours, long-distance running makes very little sense. The reality is that interval training is the best preparation for any baseball player.

Basketball

Most basketball players play pickup games whenever they aren't in-season. So their off-season training should augment the conditioning they are getting on the court and ensure the knees and ankles aren't getting stressed too much or too often. Therefore, I recommend bike and slide-board workouts to keep players in shape plus a lateral component with reduced pounding on the lower extremity joints.

Ice Hockey

Ice hockey has changed from a sport like football that has a very distinct off-season to a sport like basketball that has almost no off-season. Although games stop, more and more players stay on skates for a large portion of the summer with power skating and off-season tournaments. I like our hockey athletes to run in the off-season to get them out of the "skater's crouch" and lengthen the anterior hips. However, I do not have them run and skate on the same days in the off-season, so we end up doing more bike work than I like.

Keep hockey players off spin-type bikes that feed the flexion posture of the sport. I love the Airdyne and Assault AirBikes for hockey because resistance is

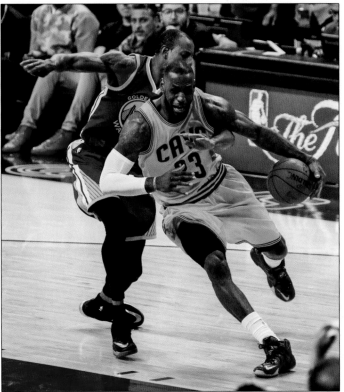

Bike and slide-board workouts keep basketball players in shape plus add a lateral component needed for the movements of their sport.

automatically adjusted, they add an upper body component to the workout (similar to running and skating), and they encourage a more upright posture.

Soccer

Aerobic training for most soccer players, particularly young, developing players, is counterproductive. Soccer players are notorious for focusing on fitness at the expense of speed. Although this approach may appear to work at the elite level, it should be noted that elite players already have world-class speed and skills. The assumption that the fitness-over-speed approach can work with younger players is both erroneous and counterproductive.

The information in this book can help soccer players and soccer coaches develop the important skills of speed and change of direction that separate the great from the near great. Soccer players need to develop fitness through tempo running and shuttle running, not jogging. The key to developing great soccer players is to develop sprinters. Coaches must understand that the training does not need to look like the testing.

Wrestling and Combat Sports

Conditioning for wrestling and other combat sports can be complicated due to the intense nature of the practices. Often these sports come with weight requirements and athletes will attempt to use exercise instead of diet to reduce to the required weight. In addition these sports are relatively unique in that the rest between periods is less than the period itself. This is referred to as a negative rest to work ratio. Combat sport athletes will obtain the majority of their conditioning through the actual practice and should be judicious in the use of additional conditioning to "make weight".

Multisport High School Athletes

Multisport athletes should follow an off-season running program if they have a season off. Rarely do athletes compete in more than two sports, so they should have at least one true off-season. However, most high school athletes continue to play the preferred sport year round. These athletes need a proper balance of rest and work during the time of year they aren't in a competitive season. But such athletes are usually highly motivated and always active. That's why I always tell coaches to ask the athletes, "What else are you planning to do today?"

CONDITIONING CONCLUSIONS

Most sports have far more similarities than differences. There are obvious differences, but what most sports have in common are the key skills of acceleration, deceleration, and change of direction. Whether you are a football player or a figure skater, these skills are critical. To improve conditioning while reducing the chance of injury, conditioning programs must train acceleration, deceleration, and change of direction. In addition, you must think outside the box. Slide boards and weight vests are two not-so-obvious tools that help make conditioning programs both sport specific and, more important, movement specific.

The following movement tables demonstrate how the nonstrength-training portion of the workout is organized.

REFERENCES

Poliquin, C. 1988. Variety in strength training. *Science Periodical on Research and Technology in Sport.* 8 (8): 1-7.

Table 11.10 Summer Movement Phase 1

Linear movement (days 1 and 3)	Lateral movement (days 2 and 4)
ROLL AND BREATHE (10 EACH SIDE)	
Glutes and hip rotators	Glutes and hip rotators
Hamstrings	Hamstrings
Calves	Calves
Lower and upper back	Lower and upper back
Posterior shoulder	Posterior shoulder
Adductors and quads	Adductors and quads
Supine knees-bent breathing	Supine knees-bent breathing
STRETCH CIRCUIT (5 BREATHS EACH SIDE)	
90/90 hip external and internal rotation	90/90 hip external and internal rotation
Box hip flexor	Box hip flexor
Adductor rock	Adductor rock
Alternating Spiderman	Alternating Spiderman
CORRECTIVES (10 EACH SIDE)	
Quadruped T-spine rotation	Supine floor slide
Leg lower	Leg lower
ACTIVATION	
Cook hip lifts (3×3) (10-second hold)	Cook hip lift (3×3) (10-second hold)
Mini-band external and internal rotation (5 each side)	Mini-band walk (10 each side)
Mini-band squat (10×)	—
MOVEMENT PREP	
Bear crawl	Half-kneeling ankle mob 10 each side
Inchworm	Body-weight squat
Knee hug	Split squat with 5-second isometric hold (5 each side)
Leg cradle	Lateral squat (5 each side)
Reverse lunge to hamstring stretch	Rotational squat (5 each side)
Single-leg straight-leg deadlift (5 each side)	Single-leg straight-leg deadlift (5 each side)
MOVEMENT SKILLS	
Straight-leg walk	Lateral march
Straight-leg skip	Lateral skip
High-knee run	Cross-behind skip
Butt kick	Cross-in-front skip
High-knee march	Shuffle
Linear skip (20 yards)	Carioca
—	Lateral crawl

Linear movement (days 1 and 3)		Lateral movement (days 2 and 4)	
Speed (4 each side)		**Ladder (day 2)**	
Day 1	Half-kneeling sprint	Shuffle wide + stick, forward and back	
Day 3	Lean, fall, and run	Cross-in-front, forward and back	
		Cross-behind, forward and back	
		In–in–out–out, forward and back	
		Scissors, right and left	
		Ladder (day 4) 3× each way	
		Crossover stick	
PLYOMETRICS			
Day 1	Box jump, 3×5	Day 2	1-leg low hurdle hop, 3×3 right and left (medial-lateral)
Day 3	1-leg hurdle hop, 3×5 right and left	Day 4	Lateral bound with stick, 3×5 each side
MEDICINE BALL			
Standing chest pass, 3×10		Standing overhead throw, 3×10 (top x on wall)	
Standing overhead slam, 3×10		Standing side toss, 3×5 each side	
AFTER LIFT			
Sled (7-8 sec)		**Conditioning**	
Days 1+3	Hard sled march (10 yd) 4/5/6 (total)	Sled crossover 2/3/3 (down and back)	
Day 1	Turf tempo run 10/12/14		
Day 3	Turf tempo run 10/12/14	Slide board 20 touch 6/7/8	
	Coach up turn	Assault bike 1 mile	

Table 11.11 Summer Movement Phase 2

Linear movement (days 1 and 3)	Lateral movement (days 2 and 4)
ROLL AND BREATHE (10 EACH SIDE)	
Glutes and hip rotators	Glutes and hip rotators
Hamstrings	Hamstrings
Calves	Calves
Lower and upper back	Lower and upper back
Posterior shoulder	Posterior shoulder
Adductors and quads	Adductors and quads
Supine knees-bent breathing	Supine knees-bent breathing
STRETCH CIRCUIT (5 BREATHS EACH SIDE)	
90/90 hip external and internal rotation	90/90 hip external and internal rotation
Box hip flexor	Box hip flexor
Adductor rock	Adductor rock
Alternating Spiderman	Alternating Spiderman
CORRECTIVES (10 EACH SIDE)	
Quadruped T-spine rotation	Supine floor slide
Leg lower	Leg lower
ACTIVATION	
Cook hip lift (3×3) (10-second hold)	Cook hip lift (3×3) (10-second hold)
Mini-band external and internal rotation (5 each side)	Mini-band walk (10 each side)
Mini-band squat (10×)	—
MOVEMENT PREP	
Bear crawl	Half-kneeling ankle mob (10 each side)
Inchworm	Body-weight squat (10×)
Knee hug	Split squat (5 each side)
Leg cradle	Lateral squat (5 each side)
Backward lunge walk with hamstring stretch	Rotational squat (5 each side)
Single-leg straight-leg deadlift	Single-leg straight-leg deadlift (5 each side)
MOVEMENT SKILLS	
Straight-leg walk	Lateral skip
Straight-leg skip	Cross-behind skip
High knee run	Cross-in-front skip
Butt kick (with knees)	Shuffle
High knee march	Carioca
Linear skip 20 yards	Lateral crawl

Linear movement (days 1 and 3)		Lateral movement (days 2 and 4)	
Speed (2/3/4 each side)		**Ladder (day 2)**	
Day 1	2-point start	Shuffle quick + stick, forward and back	
Day 3	Ball drop	1-2-3 step, forward and back	
		Crossover stick, forward and back	
		Lat in–in–out–out, forward and back	
		Scissors, right and left	
		Ladder (day 4)	
		Crossover stick to sprint	
PLYOMETRICS			
Day 1	Hurdle jump and stick, 3×5	Day 2	1-leg low hurdle hop, 3×3 R+L (medial-lateral) with mini-bounce
Day 3	1-leg hurdle hop with mini-bounce, 3×5 right and left	Day 4	45-degree bound with stick, 3×5 right and left
MEDICINE BALL			
Standing chest pass, 3×10		Staggered overhead throw, 3×5 each side (top X on wall)	
Standing overhead slam, 3×10		Stepping side toss, 3×5 each side	
AFTER LIFT			
Sled (7-8 sec)		**Conditioning**	
Days 1+3	Hard sled march, (10 yards) 6 (total)	Sled crossover, 3 (down and back)	
Day 1	150-yard shuttle 3/4/5	Slide board 30-60 sec 6/7/8	
	Coach up turn		
Day 3	Turf tempo run 12/14/16	Assault bike 1 mile	

Table 11.12 Summer Movement Phase 3

Linear movement (days 1 and 3)	Lateral movement (days 2 and 4)
ROLL AND BREATHE (10 EACH SIDE)	
Glutes and hip rotators	Glutes and hip rotators
Hamstrings	Hamstrings
Calves	Calves
Lower and upper back	Lower and upper back
Posterior shoulder	Posterior shoulder
Adductors and quads	Adductors and quads
Supine knees-bent breathing	Supine knees-bent breathing
STRETCH CIRCUIT (5 BREATHS EACH SIDE)	
90/90 Hip external and internal rotation	90/90 hip external and internal rotation
Box hip flexor	Box hip flexor
Adductor rock	Adductor rock
Alternating Spiderman	Alternating Spiderman
CORRECTIVE (10 EACH SIDE)	
Quadruped T-spine rotations	Supine floor slide
Leg lower	Leg lower
ACTIVATION	
Cook hip lift (3×3) (10-second hold)	Cook hip lift (3×3) (10-second hold)
Mini-band external and internal rotation (5 each side)	Mini-band walk (10 each side)
Mini-band squat (10×)	—
MOVEMENT PREP	
Bear crawl	Half-kneeling ankle mob (10 each side)
Inchworm	Body-weight squat (10×)
Knee hug	Forward lunge (5 each side)
Leg cradle	Lateral lunge (5 each side)
Backward lunge walk with hamstring stretch	Rotational lunge (5 each side)
Single-leg straight-leg deadlift	Single-leg straight-leg deadlift (5 each side)
MOVEMENT SKILLS	
Straight-leg walk	Lateral skip
Straight-leg skip	Cross-behind skip
High-knee run	Cross-in-front skip
Butt kick	Shuffle
High-knee march	Carioca
Linear skip (20 yards)	Lateral crawl

Linear movement (days 1 and 3)		Lateral movement (days 2 and 4)	
Speed (2/3/4 each side)		**Ladder (day 2)**	
Day 1	Plate sprint	Shuffle quick + stick, forward and back	
Day 3	Partner chase	1-2-3 cross, forward and back	
		Hip switch, forward and back	
		Crossover, forward and back	
		Scissors, right and left	
		Ladder (day 4)	
		Crossover to sprint	
PLYOS			
Day 1	—	Day 2	Single-leg low hurdle hop, 3×3 right and left (medial-lateral)
Day 3	—	Day 4	45-degree bound with mini-bounce, 3×5 each side
MEDICINE BALL			
—		Stepping overhead throw, 3×5 each side (top X on wall)	
—		Stepping side toss, 3×5 each side	
AFTER LIFT			
Sled (7-8 sec)		**Conditioning**	
Days 1+3	Sled sprint, 6×	Sled crossover, 3× (down and back)	
Day 1	300-yard shuttle, 2/3/3	Slide board, 30-60 sec 6/7/8	
	150-yard shuttle, 1/0/1	Assault bike, 1 mile	
Day 3	Turf tempo run, 16×		

Table 11.13 Summer Movement Phase 4

Linear movement (days 1 and 3)	Lateral movement (days 2 and 4)
ROLL/BREATHE (10 EACH SIDE)	
Glutes and hip rotators	Glutes and hip rotators
Hamstrings	Hamstrings
Calves	Calves
Lower and upper back	Lower and upper back
Posterior shoulder	Posterior shoulder
Adductors and quads	Adductors and quads
Supine knees bent breathing	Supine knees bent breathing
STRETCH CIRCUIT (5 BREATHS EACH SIDE)	
90/90 Hip external and internal rotators	90/90 hip external and internal rotators
Box hip flexor	Box hip flexor
Adductor rock	Adductor rock
Alternating Spiderman	Alternating Spiderman
CORRECTIVES (10 EACH SIDE)	
Quadruped T-spine rotation	Supine floor slide
Leg lower	Leg lower
ACTIVATION	
Cook hip lift (3×3) (10-second hold)	Cook hip lift (3×3) (10-second hold)
Mini-band external and internal rotation (5 each side)	Mini-band walk (10 each side)
Mini-band squat (10×)	—
MOVEMENT PREP	
Bear crawl	Half-kneeling ankle mob (10 each side)
Inchworm	Body-weight squat (10×)
Knee hug	Forward lunge (5 each side)
Leg cradle	Lateral lunge (5 each side)
Reverse lunge to hamstring stretch	Rotational lunge (5 each side)
Single-leg stiff-leg deadlift	Single-leg stiff-leg deadlift (5 each side)
MOVEMENT SKILLS	
Straight-leg walk	Lateral skip
Straight-leg skip	Cross-behind skip
High-knee run	Cross-in-front skip
Butt kick	Shuffle
High-knee march	Carioca
Linear skip (20 yards)	Lateral crawl

Linear movement (days 1 and 3)		Lateral movement (days 2 and 4)	
Speed (2/3/4 each side)		**Ladder (day 2)**	
Day 1	Plate sprint	Shuffle quick + stick, forward and back	
Day 3	Push-up start	1-2-3 cross, forward and back	
		Hip switch, forward and back	
		Lat in-in-out-out forward and back	
		Scissors reach-behind right and left	
		Ladder (day 4)	
		Crossover sprint and return	
PLYOS			
Day 1	Continuous hurdle jump (3×5)	Day 2	Single-leg low continuous hurdle hop (3×3 each side) (medial-lateral)
Day 3	Single-leg continuous hurdle hop (3×5 each side)	Day 4	Lateral bound continuous (3×5 each side)
MEDICINE BALL			
Sprinter start chest pass (3×10)		Stepping overhead throw (3×5 each side) (top X on wall)	
Standing overhead slam (3×10)		Shuffle side toss (3×5 each side)	
AFTER LIFT			
Sled (7-8 sec)		**Conditioning**	
Days 1+3	Hard sled march 10 yards 6× (total)	Sled crossover 3× down and back	
Day 1	300-yard shuttle 2/3/3	Slide board 30-60 sec 6/7/8	
	150-yard shuttle 1/0/1	Assault bike 1 mile	
Day 3	Turf tempo run 12/14/16		

Table 11.14 Winter Movement Phase 1

Breathing	Supine breathing with floor slide 10×	**Breathing**	Supine breathing w/floor slide 10×
Roll (5 each side)	Glutes + hip rotators L	**Roll (5 each side)**	Glutes + hip rotators
	Upper back		Upper back
	Low back + QL R		Low back + QL
	Posterior shoulder R		Posterior shoulder
	Adductors and quads R		Adductors and quads
Stretch circuit (20 sec each side)	Supported leg lower hamstring stretch	**Stretch circuit (20 sec each side)**	Supported leg lower hamstring stretch × 10 each side
	Box hip flexor stretch × 10 breaths (low boxes)		Box hip flexor stretch × 10 breaths (low boxes)
	Wedge hip rotator × 10 breaths		Wedge hip rotator × 10 breaths
	Active Spiderman		Active Spiderman
	Active adductor rocking with breath		Active adductor rocking with breath
Activation	Bilateral hip lift 3 × 10-sec holds (exhale out air)	**Mobility**	Standing ankle mobs × 10 each side
	Mini-band circuit ER isometric hold R/L/BI × 10 sec + 10 reps		Leg swings × 15 each side
	SL holds 2 × 10 sec each side (no band)		Isometric split squat 5 + 5 split squat
Active Warm-up (Focus on skip coaching and sprint coaching)	Bear crawl		Lateral squat × 5 each side
	Inchworm	**Add hip hinge**	Rotational squat × 5 each side
	Lateral bear crawl		Single-leg deadlift × 8 each side
	Knee to chest	**Active warm-up**	March to high-knee skip
	Leg cradle		Lateral skip
	Heel to butt		Cross-in-front skip
	Single-leg deadlift with reach		Cross-behind skip
	Backward lunge walk with hamstring stretch		Side shuffle
	March to high knee skip		Carioca
	Lateral skip		Lateral crawl
	High knee run	**Ladder**	Shuffle wide + stick F/B
	Heel-ups		Cross in front F/B
	Straight-leg walk		Cross behind F/B
	Straight-leg skip		In-in-out-out F/B
	Backpedal		Scissors R/L
	Backward run		
Speed (Use wall drills for younger athletes that do not understand hip separation, 3×5 each side.)	Lean, fall, and run × 3 each side		

Plyo	Day 1: Box jump: 3×5	**Plyo**	Day 1: Single-leg medial/lateral low hurdle hop: 3×3 each side
	Day 2: Single-leg ladder/low hurdle hop: 3×5		Day 2: Lateral bound in place with stick: 3×5 each side
Medicine ball	Medicine ball overhead throw: 3×10	**Medicine ball**	Medicine ball overhead throw: 3×10
	Medicine ball side toss: 3×10 each side		Medicine ball side toss: 3×10 each side
Conditioning	Treadmill tempo runs: ×8, ×10, ×12 Increase incline before speed; speed never above 10.0	**Conditioning**	Tempo runs (same as day 1)
	Beginners/Regression: mat runs/ walk on the treadmill if enough turf space		Explosive slide board × 20 total touches ×3, ×4, ×5 sets (coach 1 rep at a time)

INDEX

Note: The italicized *f* and *t* following page numbers refer to figures and tables, respectively.

ABOUT THE AUTHOR

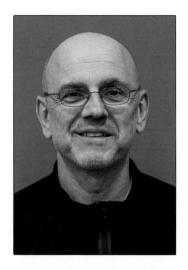

Michael Boyle is one of the foremost experts in the fields of strength and conditioning, functional training, and general fitness. He is known internationally for his pioneering work and is an in-demand speaker at strength and conditioning conferences and athletic training clinics around the world.

Because of his expertise in sport performance training, Boyle has coached elite athletes on teams such as the Boston Red Sox, Boston Bruins, New England Revolution, and Boston Breakers as well as the U.S. women's Olympic teams in soccer and ice hockey. In 2012, Boyle joined the Boston Red Sox coaching staff as a strength and conditioning consultant for the team, which later won the World Series.

His client list over the years reads like a Who's Who of athletic success, including retired American football defensive end Marcellus Wiley, 2012 Olympic judo gold medalist Kayla Harrison, and Liverpool striker Daniel Sturridge.

Boyle was the head strength and conditioning coach at Boston University from 1984 to 1997. From 1990 to 2012 he was the strength and conditioning coach for men's ice hockey at BU.

Boyle provides performance-enhancement training for athletes of all levels through his Boston-based gym, Mike Boyle Strength and Conditioning, which has been named one of America's 10 Best Gyms by *Men's Health* magazine. Boyle's range of experience includes training athletes from the middle school level to all-stars in most major professional sports.

Boyle is the owner and editor of StrengthCoach.com, a website dedicated to educating strength and conditioning coaches and personal trainers.

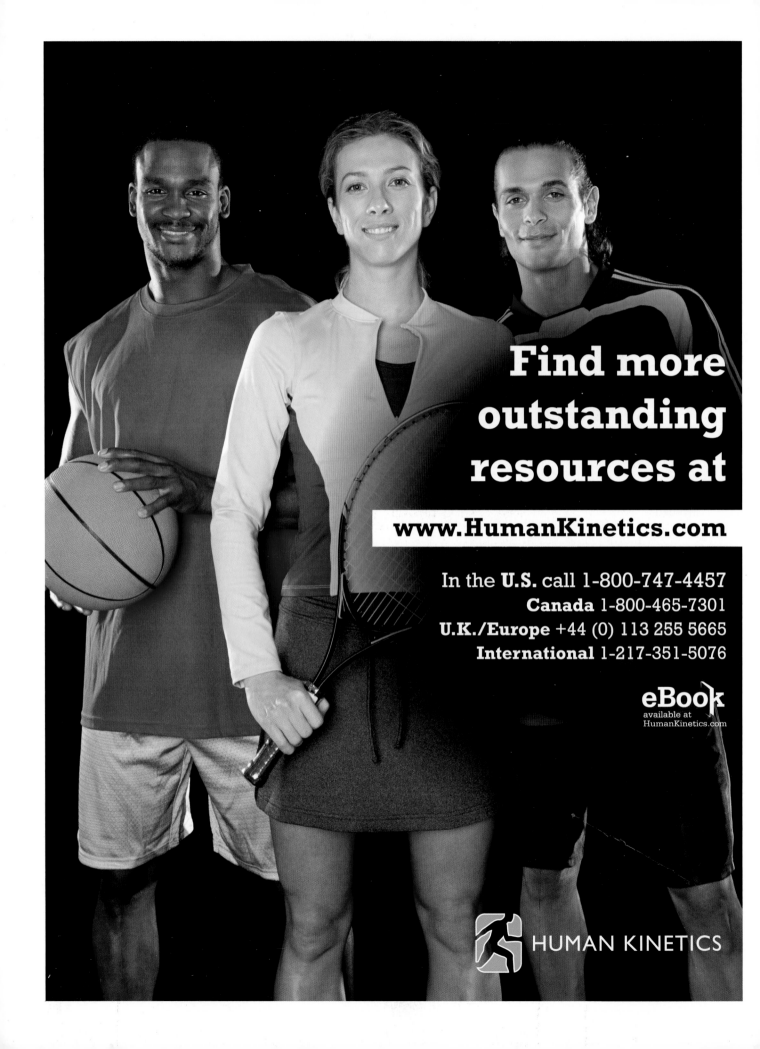